CW01649153

Holding Mama

A RESOURCE JOURNAL FOR THE THIRD AND FOURTH TRIMESTERS

Dedicated to

Peter and Daniel, Sienna and Kolbe
for making us mamas

Clare and Danielle
for being the mamas to hold us

For international orders, please find our ebook and hardcopy on Amazon.com or visit www.holdingmama.co.za. First edition self-published in 2021.

Copyright Caitlin Scott and Caryn Edwards.

No parts of this book may be reproduced in any form or by any means without the prior written permission of the authors.

Paperback ISBN 978-1-991206-16-9
E-Book ISBN 978-1-991206-17-6

Contents

INTRODUCTION

PART ONE | THE THIRD TRIMESTER

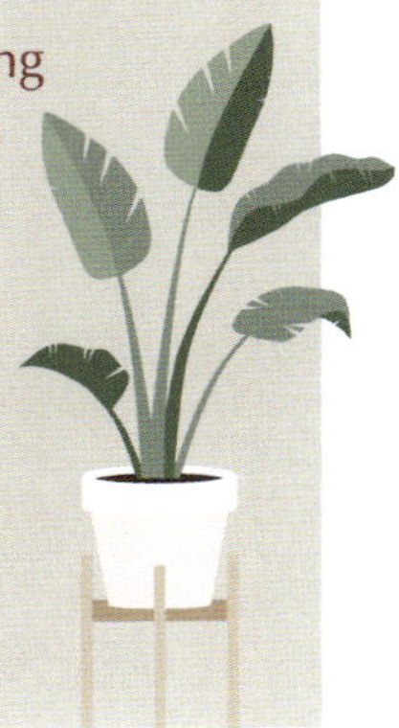

Contents

PART TWO | THE FOURTH TRIMESTER

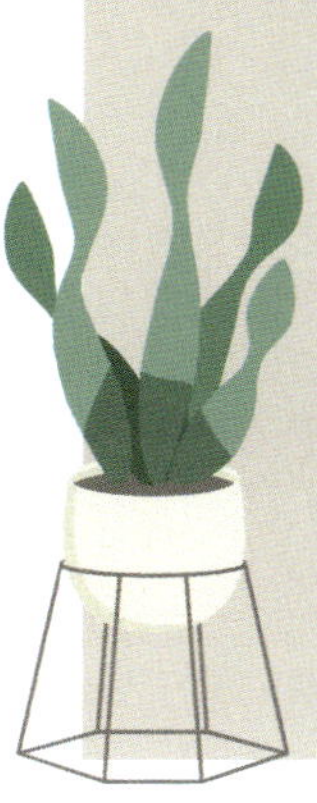

Contents

PART THREE | WEEKLY REFLECTIONS

A JOURNALLING CHAPTER

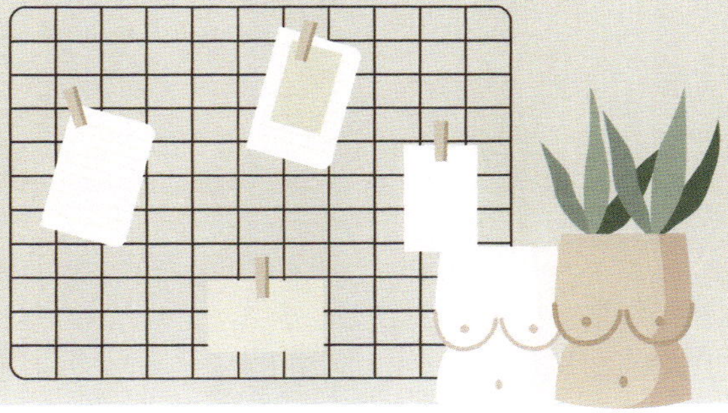

FOREWORD

Motherhood is a journey and adventure like no other and, like all journeys, it brings with it challenges, anxieties and then moments of absolute joy and splendour!

By writing this book, Caryn and Caitlin have not only created a guide for mothers with reference to their words of experience and wisdom, but they have also given mothers the voice of a caring friend. The cathartic style and content of *Holding Mama* provides comfort and support through the early days and beyond.

As a specialist paediatrician, I have seen many first time mothers grapple with the changes that naturally occur in their daily routines, their relationship with their spouses and their relationship with themselves. As a mother, I have personally gone through these trials and tribulations and understand fully that no matter how prepared you may think you are, motherhood is a journey of transformation of mind, body and soul that you can never be fully prepared for.

This book stands out in the way in which it confronts all those changes from the third to fourth trimester and provides new mums with the necessary tools and words of wisdom to help them through those days, weeks and months of transition - many of which will be a toolbox for life. From the weekly planners that remind new mothers to make time for peace, joy and rest whilst tackling their weekly routines, to journaling questions offering moments of reflection and introspection, to guidance on birth choices, postpartum care, feeding choices, sleeping, bonding and so much more, this book could be considered as the ultimate handbook, guide and companion that every mum should have.

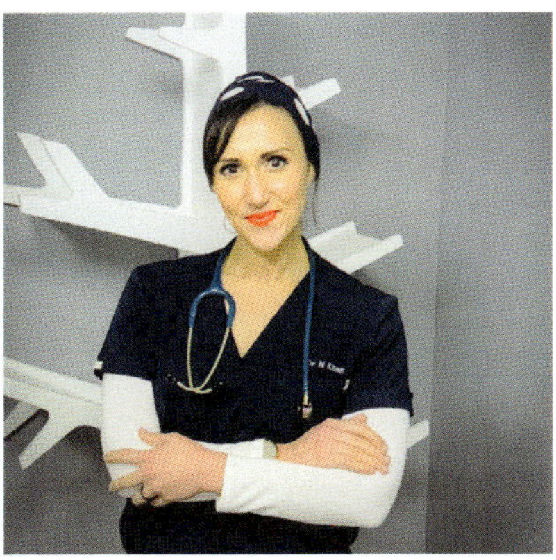

Dr Nadia Khan is a mum and paediatrician based in Hillcrest, KwaZulu Natal. Dr Khan's approach to treatment is holistic and her main goal is to promote optimal health for all children through prevention of disease and appropriate treatment when signs of illness occur.

You will find her at www.drnadiakhan.co.za and you can follow her on Instagram: @dr.nadia.khan

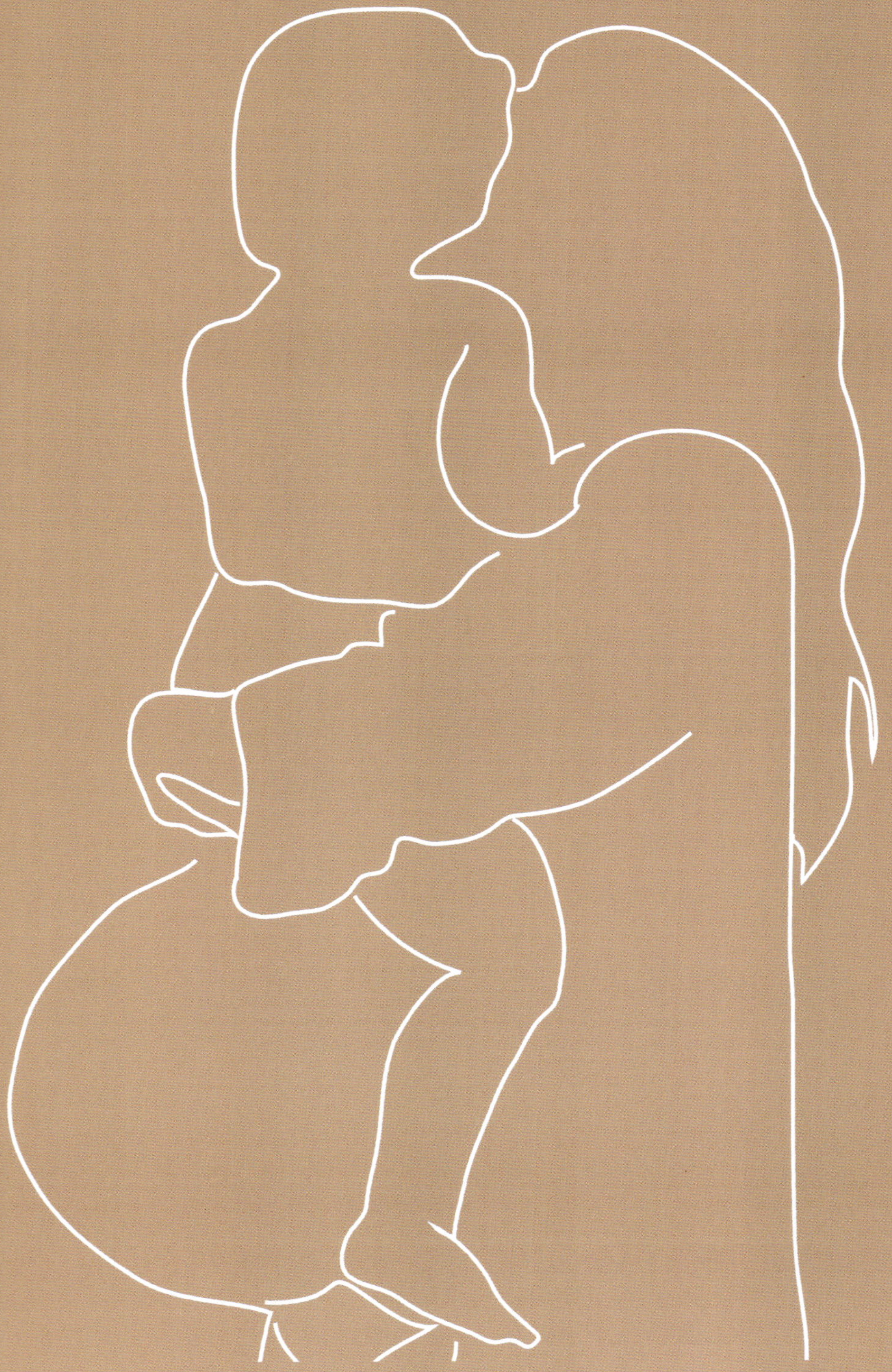

Hello, mama.

PREFACE

Three years ago, our motherhood journeys crossed. What started out as a friendship over coffee and soulful conversation grew into voice notes and messages around motherhood. Revealed musings: how unprepared we had felt in becoming mothers and why a lot of what went on in our bodies, minds and souls was often considered taboo. Why had we felt so unprepared? Why had no one told us before we became mothers? Why was it so difficult, at times, to talk about these topics with fellow mums?

While both of us had supportive friends, we were not immune to the loneliness that so many mothers encounter. The proverbial phrase "it takes a village to raise a child" has become a foreign and idealistic concept in today's society, where many mothers are raising children from a place that feels like they are alone.

What became a more pressing question on our minds was 'where is the *village* to hold Mum'? Antenatal classes often prepare mums-to-be to take care of the practical sides of birthing a child, but do little to equip mums in navigating their own changing identities, the new role assumed and the challenges that are presented to our minds, bodies and souls.

We believe that when a mum is in touch with what is going on within, she is able to experience a deeper freedom. By recognising her own physical and emotional needs, she will unearth a strength she never knew possible, as she grows into her new identity by being honest about where she is at.

We will be sharing tools which will help you embrace your circumstances when no one is there to hold you; and to harness the gift of vulnerability that will enable you to share in the collective joys and struggles common to mums all around the world.

We deeply hope that this journal will be a road for you to access a village of support. May our stories spark the reassurance of knowing that you are not alone, that you are enough and that you have your own story in the making.

“

The proverbial phrase, 'It takes a village to raise a child', has become a foreign and idealistic concept in today's society, where many mothers are raising children from a place that feels like they are alone.

What became a more pressing question on our minds was, **'where is the *village* to hold Mum'?**

”

Meet the authors

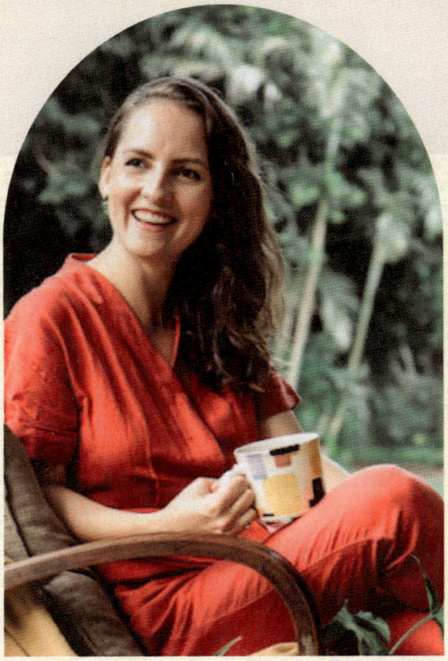

Caryn

Caryn is a life coach who has a special interest in coaching teenagers, mothers and adults seeking direction in life. Her life coaching approach is focused on one's way of being - to shift one's reality on the holistic level of mood, body and language. These three threads of her coaching are woven through the journaling section. Caryn is wife to Steven, mama to Sienna and Kolbe and lives in Hillcrest, South Africa. Coffee, croissants and writing (preferably combined together) are what fuel her motherhood journey.

“

I raised her. But in many ways, she raised me...

”

"I suppose the only babies I encountered were those I saw from afar - the ones sound asleep in prams and coffee shops. I am the last born so I didn't know how to handle a baby, yet I knew I wanted a handful to mother one day. My pregnancy was smooth and I basked in the glow of nurturing an unknown life and dreaming of the girl she might be.

When I did meet her - bright eyed, craning her strong neck - I was in awe of her beauty. She slept the first day when all the visitors came and then the visitors left and I felt alone and unequipped to deal with an unsettled baby who seemed to always be hungry - a hunger I felt I couldn't satisfy on many levels. I felt let down by the illusion of idyllic motherhood, I doubted my instincts and I wondered if and when I would ever find joy and integration again... Why did no one tell me it would be this hard? That newborn I struggled with is now my beloved toddler who fills my eyes with awe each day - the way she prattles on with exquisite language and endless energy and charm. I raised her, but in many ways, she's raised me - raised in me love and strength, providing a toolkit of learning and unlearning with her unique blueprint, the one not written in the books but forged between her and me.

I am now a mother of a sweet boy, and I have found this second round of parenting to be soaked with a deeper trust in my instincts; holding the phases lightly, with the perspective that the tricky bits always pass.

I am so thankful for this journey of motherhood; and I hope that what we have written, the lessons we have lived, will widen your hope for all that motherhood has in store for you."
- Caryn, *Life Shifts Coaching*

LIFE SHIFTS
COACHING
with Cary

FIND CARYN ONLINE AT
instagram.com/life_shifts_coaching
www.lifeshiftscoaching.co.za

Meet the authors

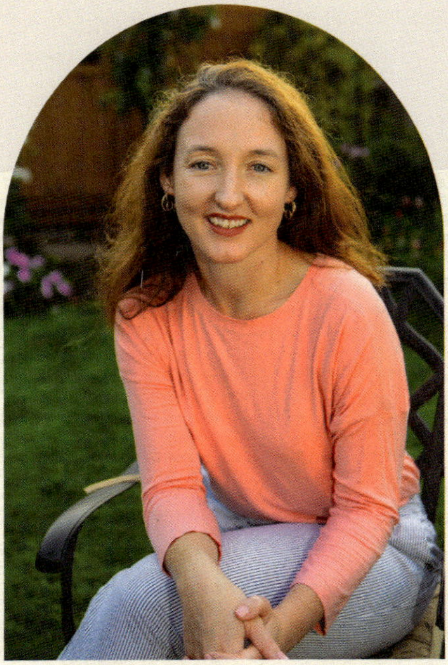

Caitlin

Caitlin is a medical doctor with a passion for women's health and holistic medicine. She works at a private GP practice with a focus on preventing illness through health optimisation using nutritional as well as regenerative medicine. She has a number of years of experience with intravenous iron and vitamin infusions to treat nutritional deficiencies as well as body identical hormone therapy to treat PMS, PCOS and peri-menopausal symptoms. Caitlin is wife to David, mum to Peter and Daniel and lives in Hertfordshire, United Kingdom. Conversations, coffee and cuddles are what fuel her motherhood journey.

"

It takes time and a gentle realistic expectation of what is possible and what can be 'let go'.

"

THE MEWS PRACTICE

PRIVATE GENERAL PRACTITIONERS
&
REGENERATIVE MEDICINE CLINIC

"I always wanted to be a mum. I grew up as a little girl that loved spending time with people and wanting to do what I could to make them happy. This translated into studying medicine and starting my career with a deep passion for women and my mission to help them find contentment. I spent time working with babies as a medical officer in a neonatal hospital and as a GP in a women's health practice.

Then I discovered that I was pregnant with our first son. I thought that my medical experience, my deep desire for motherhood and my calm nature would make me immune to the difficulties that other mothers experienced. So you can imagine my confusion when I sat alone in the dark cold night, crying with exhaustion, trying to rock my baby to sleep. Those first six months were hard. I mostly did not know what to do. I constantly questioned if what I was doing was right. Was I being indulgent? Was I spoiling my child? Was I teaching him bad habits?

What was more confusing was the opinions that others so readily shared on how best to do things. It was the apparent ease with which they seemed to navigate the challenges that I found quite tough. Through experience, I found that I was different to any other mum, and my son was different to any other baby, so our combination was unique and we would both need to learn together, as in any other new role that life presents.

When my second son was born just twenty months after my first, I realized this all over again, together with the challenges of a not yet two year old. It takes time and a gentle realistic expectation of what is possible and what can be 'let go'."
- Caitlin, *The Mews Practice*

FIND CAITLIN ONLINE AT
www.themewspractice.com

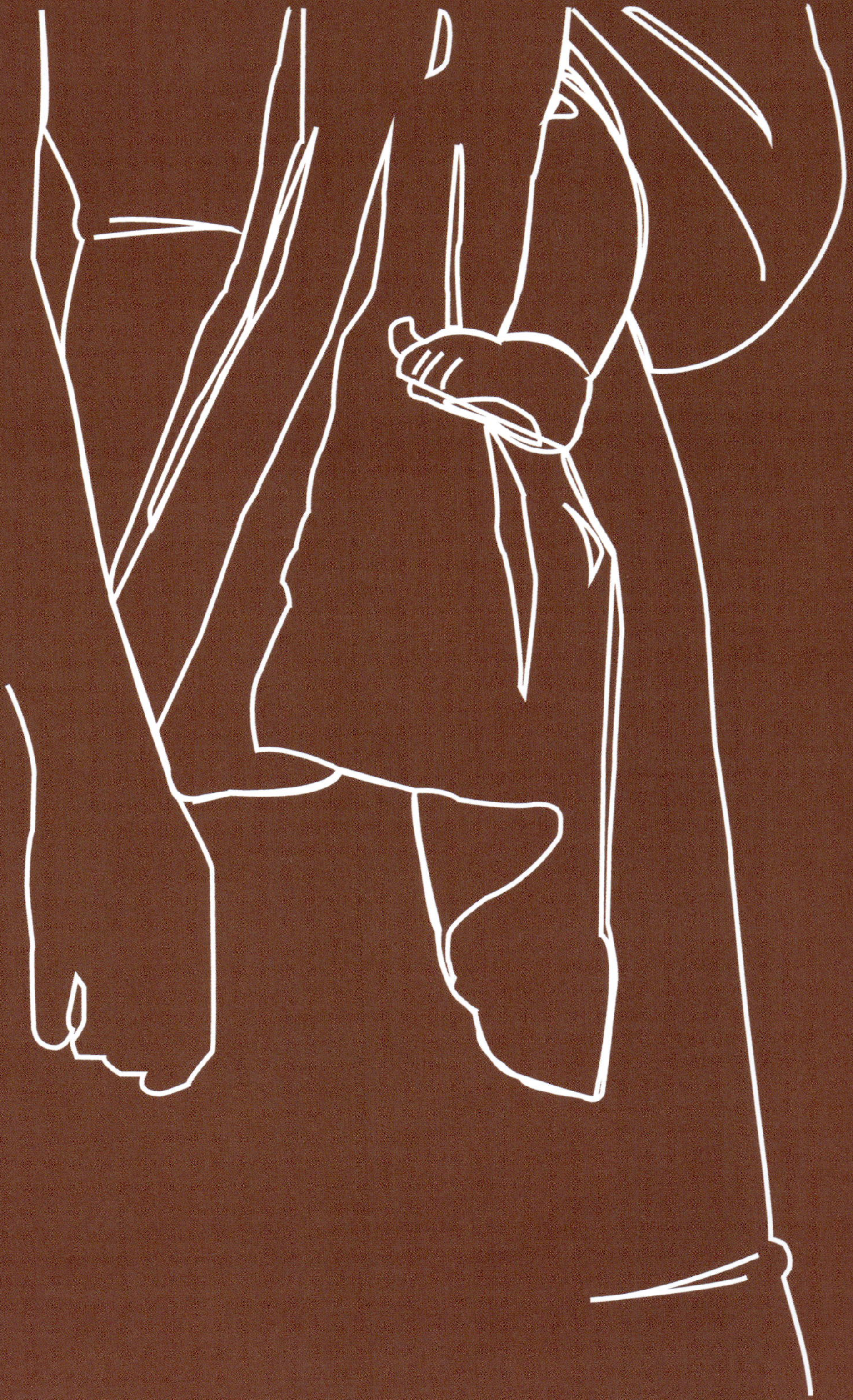

Guest contributors

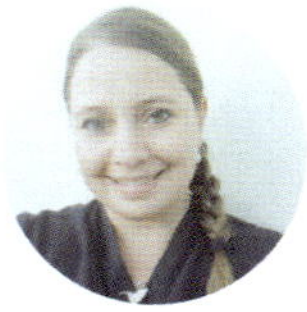

Charlene Yared West is a Doula, Hypnotherapist, Hypnobirthing practitioner and founder of Relax Into Birth Online Hypnobirthing, based in Cape Town South Africa. She is Mum to Leonardo.
You can find her online at www.relaxintobirth.com.

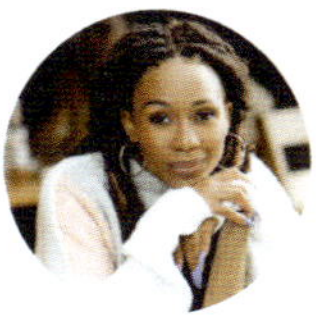

Dr Mpume Zenda is an OB-GYN-Sexologist, based in South Africa. She is passionate about sexual and reproductive health; and being a part of such conversations both as a woman and clinician. Her hope for you as a new mom is that you would feel seen, heard and supported through this book and that you would be patient with yourself as your body changes through this beautiful, but sometimes painful and frustrating process. Dr. Zenda's practice is based in Morningside, Johannesburg. You can follow her on Instagram @dr.gynae.

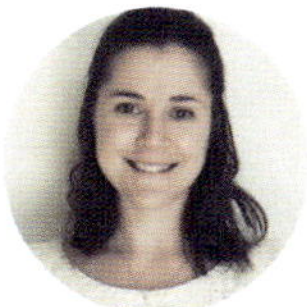

Jen Wareing is a Women's Health Physio and is a mother of two small children, Lily and Cooper. She has a passion for empowering expectant and new mums with knowledge, which will help them navigate this season in their lives and help them find hope, healing and support. Follow her on Facebook and instagram: physio_beyondthebump to learn helpful tips along your journey. Jen lives in KwaZulu Natal, South Africa.

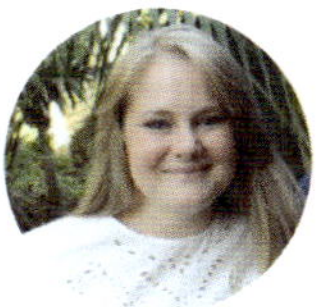

Holly Peretz is a Pediatric Occupational Therapist, toddler mom and the founder of otholly.com. Through her blog, online conference and membership area she aims to make early child development accessible and easy to understand for toddler mamas. Holly is passionate about making the little years fun, lighter and more colourful.

Guest contributors

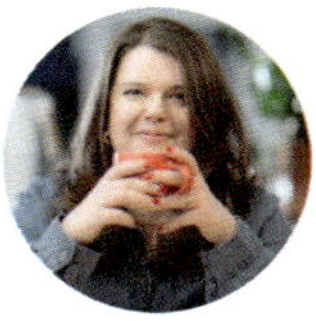

Kerry Secker is an infant sleep consultant and Founder of the Care It Out sleep approach (Care It Out). She's on a mission to support parents to a settled night sleep without sleep training. She's based in London but, through a gentle approach, has supported families to get more sleep all across the globe. You can find Kerry online at Instagram @careitoutsleepconsultant or www.careitout.com.

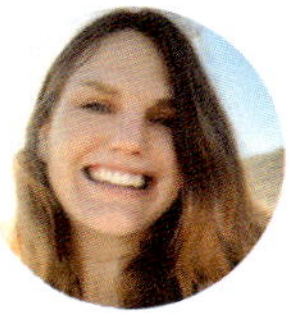

Georgie Avery is a registered nurse who now specialises in infant feeding with a specific focus on breastfeeding. She is a mom to three boys and through her own varied experiences is passionate about being a support and guide to mothers and babies, especially in those early weeks when mom and baby are discovering their own unique relationship.

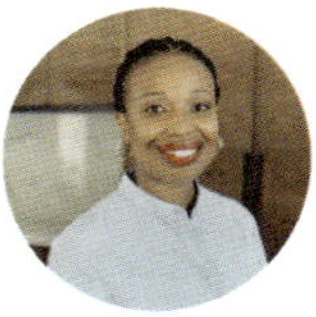

Bongi Hill is a doctor, wife to Deane and mama to two precious children, Lukhanyo and Esona. Bongi and her family live the slow farm life in Tulbagh, South Africa. She is passionate about hands-on positive parenting, nature and connecting with people. She shares her parenting journey and family adventures on her social media platform @ndibambe, which means 'hold me' in Xhosa, her home language.

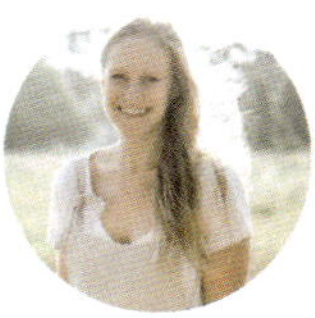

Kelly Lubbee is a graphic designer with a love for minimalist design that allows you to breathe. As a mama herself, she knows the need to take time to regroup in these early months. Her desire behind the design of this book would be that you feel a sense of calm amongst what may feel like chaos, and that you would want to truly take the time to reflect on these extremely crazy beautiful days ahead.
You can find her online through www.theselulajourney.com.

About *Holding Mama* and how to use this book

Holding Mama is designed to help prepare you for motherhood by informing you about the practical nature of topics, as well as creating a safe space where you can be held by checking in with yourself, engaging with the topics from a holistic angle and, perhaps, inspiring you to reach out to others along the way. We have tried to present information honestly and conversationally as we would chat with a friend with the deepest hope that you will turn to your instincts to guide you.

The journaling activities throughout the book utilise self-coaching as a tool to empower you by helping you search within for answers. The chapters have been named to allow you to 'dip-in' whenever you feel challenged or inspired to do so. Don't feel restricted by the topics - rather look for ones that match your stage in your motherhood journey. The book has been designed as a resource journal to refer to whenever necessary. If you find that you need support along the way, we encourage you to use the tool of vulnerability which we discuss in week two of the weekly reflections and to reach out to someone, whether they are a health professional or a person you trust and can confide in.

You are welcome to contact us - we would love to hear how this book might impact you. As this book grows its reach, we hope that you will connect with other mums using it and we invite you to join our community of readers on our Facebook and Instagram page.

You will find topics signposted by the icons of 'BODY', 'MIND' and SOUL'. Most of what we face as mums is never boxed as one or the other - something physical is often simultaneously experienced more complexly in mind and soul. But we have labelled them as such so as to invite you to start engaging with topics from a holistic angle.

use these icons to guide you

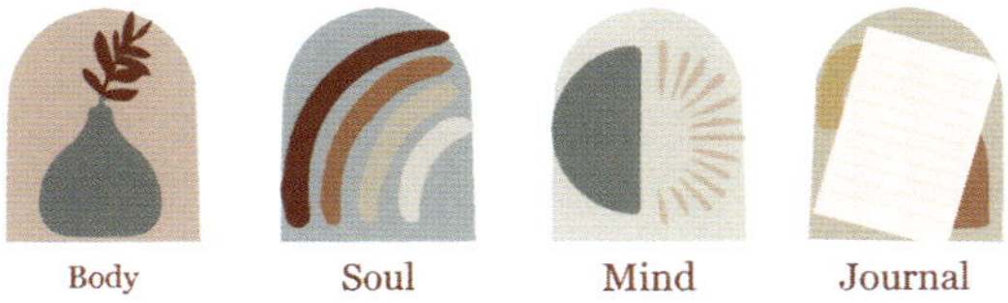

This book is divided into three parts:

The Third Trimester section is designed for you to work through at any stage of your pregnancy journey.

The Fourth Trimester is designed to equip you to navigate the shift to nurturing yourself while caring for your growing baby.

The weekly journaling is designed for you to check in with yourself each week. It offers tools for you to practise as well as a 'check-in' to see how you are doing with implementing your postpartum support plan. Don't feel pressurised to complete it during the fourth trimester - use it when you feel the need for reflection, inspiration and self-coaching.

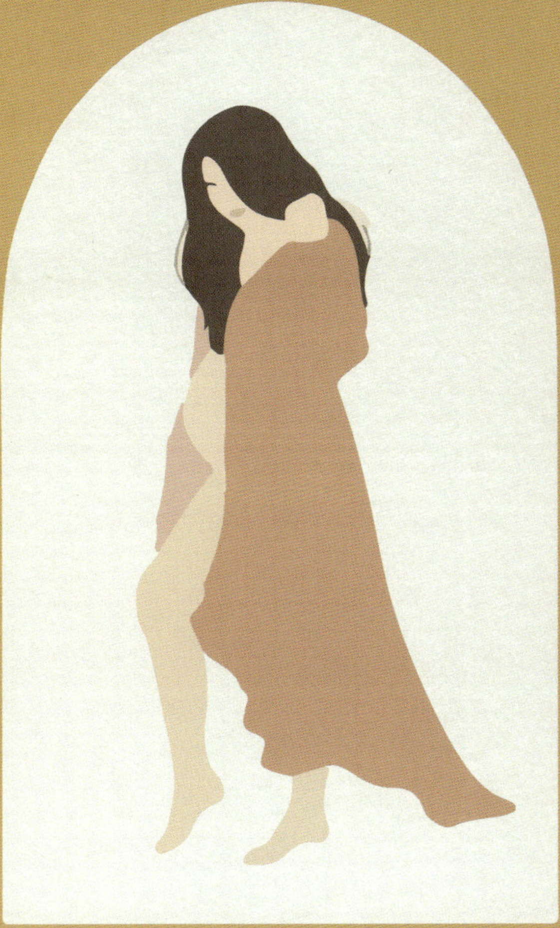

THE Third Trimester

"Everything grows rounder and wider and weirder, and I sit here in the middle of it all and wonder who in the world you will turn out to be."

- Carrie Fisher

KNOWING YOUR TRIGGERS

by Caryn

Pregnancy is certainly an emotional time, particularly in the first trimester when your body is being whacked by hormonal changes. Know that whatever emotional experience you are having is completely acceptable.

CHECK IN:

How are you feeling about your pregnancy currently? If you find it helpful, you can identify emotions and areas of both gratitude for the journey and challenges you might be experiencing. Without having to 'fix' the challenges, simply hold space for yourself by noticing where these mind, body and soul experiences sit in your body. Let your breath expand those areas of tension and gratitude. Know that it is normal to hold contradictory emotions.

TIP:

As you experience stress, feel free to name it and write it down as a way of both acknowledging and offloading. You might find it helpful to having a running list of tasks and questions that arise during your pregnancy.

GRATITUDE	CHALLENGES & STRESSORS

UNDERSTANDING YOUR PERSONALITY TYPE:

It can be useful to spend some time learning about how your dominant personality traits respond to certain situations. What you find overwhelming or stressful may differ to what others feel anxious about. There are many tools that can assist you in identifying your strong traits and the ways in which you respond in stable and stressed states. This will aid you in understanding why certain things may trigger you and recognising those triggers will help you to feel more in control. If you have a partner, it is also helpful to know what personality type they are so that you can recognise their needs and triggers.

THE ENNEAGRAM

There are many personality tests which can help you to identify what triggers you as an individual, mother and partner.

The Enneagram is a helpful example of a personality test. The official test (which you pay for) provides an indepth analysis, but there are free tests online that could give you an indication of your type. After doing this free test and reading the descriptions of the different numbers and their wings, you might be able to decide which one you are.

It can be helpful for partners to do it too and you can read a description of your combination when in a relationship on this website.

https://www.enneagraminstitute.com/the-enneagram-type-combinations

scan the code

to visit the link

THE ENNEAGRAM IN MOTHERHOOD

by Caitlin

My dominant number is a 1 with strong 9 and 2 wings. This means I am a person that is idealistic and desperately wants to do what is right. It also means that I struggle when I can't list and measure my efforts and tick them off as being well done. As a new mother, I would get to the end of the day, feeling exhausted by the demands of the day but unable to quantify what I had actually done. I'd yearn for appreciation but would not ask for it and found that my most challenging time was when I was at home on my own with no one to see the effort I was putting into caring for my children.

by Caryn

After I did the enneagram test, I knew instinctively that I was a type 4 because I feel deeply. I am very aware of my emotional landscape and my flaws. The temptation for me is to think that my emotional experience is my reality - forever. So when I had a rocky start to motherhood, I thought that this was a telltale sign of how I would be as a mother. I felt a bit disappointed by how challenging it was in contrast to the grand ideal I had imagined it to be. Things did get easier. Now I know that I don't need to take my emotions so seriously and that phases pass. When I've bumped up against these feelings when one of my children is sick or when I've discerned how best to navigate discipline with a toddler, I've learnt to view these difficult patches with more equanimity.

Becoming aware of internal and external triggers will help you navigate this time so that you can experience a more peaceful way of being as you prepare to meet your baby. It would be wise to reach out to someone if you are battling with anxiety or need to process some of these emotional triggers. Here are a few examples of triggers that pregnant mothers can experience:

EXTERNAL TRIGGERS

- Giving birth during a pandemic
- Financial concerns
- Strained relationship with partner
- Being a single parent
- Navigating boundaries with extended family
- A lack of support from the community

INTERNAL TRIGGERS

- Fear of miscarriage
- Previous trauma
- Doubts about being a good parent
- Changes to your physical body and body image
- Changing identity
- Changing lifestyle and giving up certain 'freedoms'
- Deciding if or how you might juggle work and motherhood

It can be very helpful to examine what lies beneath the stresses that come your way during pregnancy and as you prepare to give birth. By simply acknowledging the triggers, they will have less power over you. Be encouraged to reach out for the support you might need, whether it's processing your emotions with someone or asking for help in practical areas such as getting your house ready for baby or cooking some meals to freeze (perhaps someone in your social circle can draw up a meal train for the weeks after the birth). If you would like to receive tools on how to communicate your needs, you can find more on this in the chapter of 'making requests'.

TRIGGERS IN MOTHERHOOD

by Caitlin

In my first pregnancy, I made the decision at 32 weeks to change my service provider from an Obstetrician to private midwives. As a health professional that had overseen many normal deliveries and cut many cesareans, I felt quite anxious of being forced into a premature surgery. I spent hours reading up on how to shift my baby into the correct position to engage and did so many squats and lunges that I physically hurt. Despite my efforts, my due date came and went and my baby showed no signs of being ready to make his journey out into the world. The daily messages from loved ones asking if I felt any changes or if I thought that day would be the day, made me feel like I was somehow failing before the job had even begun. The questions triggered self doubt as to whether I was capable of the monstrous task at hand.

TRIGGERS IN MOTHERHOOD

by Caryn

During my first pregnancy, I was much too caught up in a bubble of elation that I didn't experience many triggers. It was only in my second pregnancy that I began to experience some anxiety; the first being: pregnant in a pandemic. For my first birth, I was supported by a doula and private midwives in a hospital. This time around, as this was not an option where I now lived, I had to make peace with the situation that, with going into a hospital birth in a pandemic, there would be protocols that I wouldn't be comfortable with: first and foremost, would my husband be allowed to be at the birth? Secondly, would I get my COVID test in time if or when labour commenced naturally? My concerns led to some discerning conversations and, in the end, I surprised myself by opting for a home birth.

The next trigger hit me in the latter part of the third trimester as I was approaching my due date. I suddenly felt like I didn't want to give birth and that I hadn't processed that I was actually going to have another baby. I had struggled so much the first time around - why was I wanting to do this again? I wondered if I would be connected to this baby, with my focus being on my toddler during the entire pregnancy. I also realised that I feared birth more this time and started grappling with the trauma of my first birth which, perhaps, I hadn't fully processed.

I allowed fear to be present to me. As a Life Coach, I teach my clients that all emotions signpost something and we can get over them by letting ourselves pass through them - rather than running away.

So I spent some time processing my fears and it served me well. I spoke to my midwives about my fears, I journaled and wrote down what was triggering me. I wrote down birth affirmations and listened to my hypnobirthing tracks (we will discuss Hypnobirthing as a tool). I created a playlist of songs, reflecting on their meaningful lyrics, using them as a mantra to ground me in times of fear. When I went over my due date by ten days I had established a deeper trust in my body, in my instincts and felt eager to meet my son, with whom I now have a deep connection. By releasing those fears, taking the time to journal, pray and talk with those in my support network, I felt more empowered going into birth. Processing your triggers might be uncomfortable but will be worth it in the long run.

Deep breathing is the quickest way to self-regulate. When you are stressed, your sympathetic nervous system is activated which is characterised by fight, flight or freeze mode which makes it difficult to think clearly and react calmly. The easiest way to regain calm is to breathe deeply from your diaphragm which will shift you into the parasympathetic nervous system (rest and digest mode) which is activated when you feel safe and grounded. Try it now - breathe in for 4-6 counts and out for 6-8 counts. Continue to do this, allowing the flow of air to be both natural, filling the base of your belly rather than your shoulders. Find your rhythm and notice how you feel for slowing down yourbreath. You can do this whenever you face anxiety along your motherhood journey.

scan the code

for a guided meditation on emotional triggers and where they lie in the body - by Caryn

Try not to label your emotions as positive or negative - simply observe what they are and how they might or might not be serving you.

Start by seating yourself comfortably and upright, feet grounded on the floor. You might like to close your eyes as you centre yourself. Take a deep breath. Continue to breathe as you let go of all distractions, focusing only on your breath.

Observe how your body is feeling. Without needing to fix or analyse, pinpoint any areas of tension, breathing into them. Accept the tension, focus on these areas of tension, rather than avoiding them. Notice what gentle attention does to these areas.

Now reflect on where you might be holding tension in your body with regards to any sense of concerns or triggers you may have identified as you approach motherhood. By linking where these emotions live in your body, you will be able to release the anxiety more fully.

Breathe in again for 4-6 and out for 6-8 counts until you feel more grounded. Gently bring your focus back to the room. Use this simple practice whenever you need to check in with yourself, and especially in times of stress in any stage of your parenting journey.

COMMON THIRD TRIMESTER CHALLENGES

by Caitlin

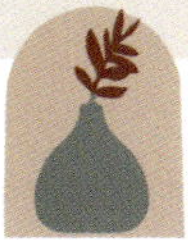

The third trimester is filled with a combination of excitement about meeting your child and exhaustion of the changed body that you fill. The physical effects of pregnancy can be very grueling which can fuel the impatience to meet your little one.

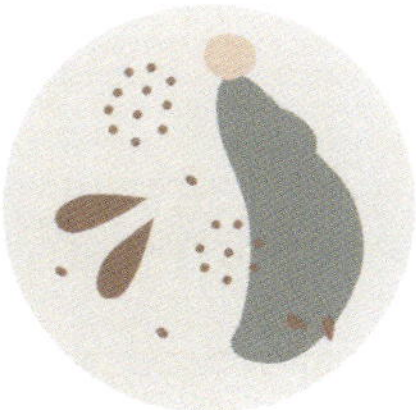

BODY ACHES

Relaxin is a hormone that is made to loosen the ligaments holding bones together. This is mainly to help accommodate your baby's head as it passes through the pelvis but it can result in lower back pain, sciatica shock-like sensations running down your leg and wrist pain. Back pain is further exacerbated by your changed sense of gravity that is carried by your pelvic floor in front of your body.

A warm bath with water, to softly hold your tummy or a hot water bottle can ease this discomfort. A chiropractor will have helpful manipulations that can ease this discomfort.

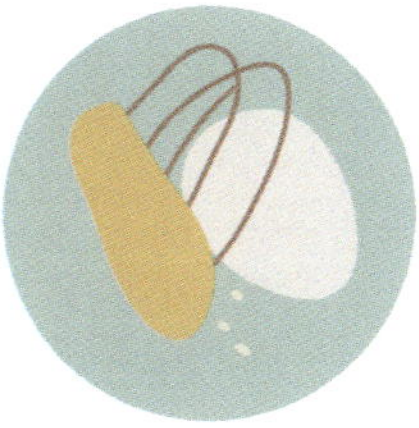

MUSCULAR SPASMS

Many women get muscle cramps or spasms that can be difficult to shift. Magnesium is wonderful at soothing aches and has the added benefit of calming these at night to help you sleep. Some people bath in magnesium salts, others use a magnesium spray and many take it at very low doses as an oral supplement before bed.

BREAST PAIN

Hormones increase glands for milk production which increases breast size. Try not to wear the same bra as you did before falling pregnant or a bra that is too tight, as it may cause back pain because of too little support. The breast compression could also suppress milk production.

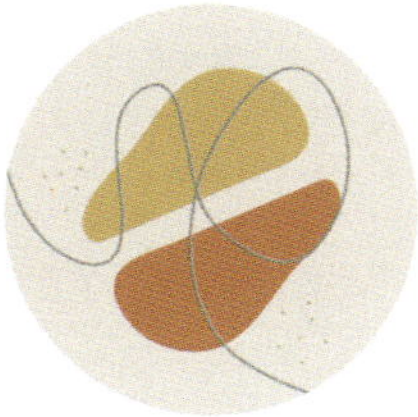

PELVIC PAIN

As your baby's head descends into the pelvis you can sometimes feel kicks against the rib end of the amniotic sac forcing their head towards the vagina. Your pelvic floor has held the weight of the placenta, fluid and baby for months and it can be normal to experience deep vaginal aches in the last weeks of pregnancy.

Pregnancy pilates is a great way to stretch those aching muscles, move to ease ligament pain and strengthen all means of support. You can also buy a support belt to help hold the weight of your tummy.

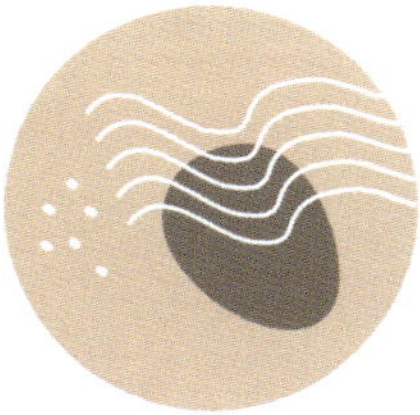

ACID REFLUX

In order to extract maximum nutrition from the food we eat when pregnant, the rate of passage through the gut slows down. This, together with the stomach being compressed against the expanding uterus, causes the dreaded heartburn from acid laden food being pressed up into the oesophagus. It is worse when lying down or even sitting. Eating smaller, more frequent meals that are creamy as opposed to spicy or acidic can help relieve the symptoms. Antacids like Gaviscon liquid used at low doses and infrequently can soothe reflux that is waking you up at night.

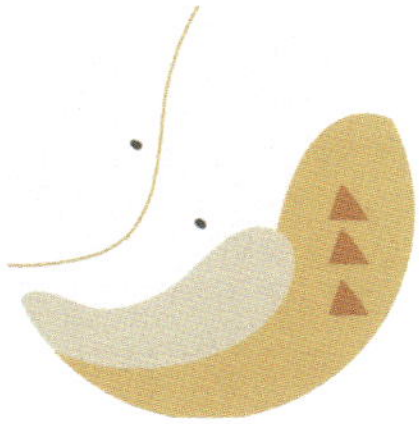

SWELLING

Your blood volume almost doubles in pregnancy and this, together with the compression of your veins carrying blood back to your heart, results in blood pooling in your legs. This causes swollen ankles but should not cause a puffy face which is something your healthcare professional will want to check. The increased blood volume and compression on the bladder makes you need to wee more too.

Try lifting your feet onto a cushion, when you can, to help get the blood efficiently back to your heart to be circulated again.

INSOMNIA

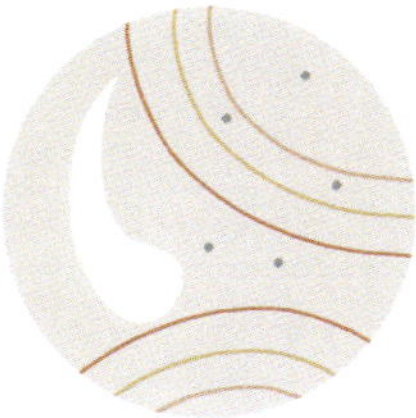

Many mothers struggle to sleep due to the difficulty to get comfortable. Try putting a breastfeeding pillow between your knees while lying on your side. Sleep troubles can be exacerbated by iron deficiency or anxiety from vitamin D deficiency. Downloading a meditation app such as Headspace or Calm or Hypnobirthing tracks can help your mind give in to sleep.

FATIGUE

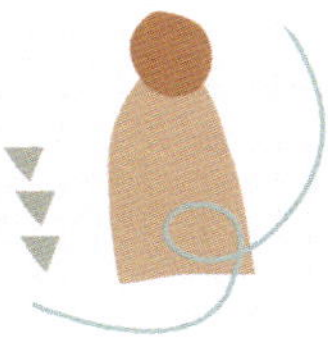

The body will divert all of your nutrients to your growing baby and in the last trimester the baby grows only in size. Iron, vitamin B12 and folate, when deficient, can all cause fatigue and brain fog. Dizziness can be related to iron or vitamin D deficiency and low blood pressure. Make sure that you are taking antenatal supplements, drinking enough water and that you get up slowly from sitting to standing.

RESTLESS LEGS

The sensation that your legs move, particularly at night, without your control can be linked to iron deficiency, vitamin B12 deficiency or vitamin D deficiency.

SEX DRIVE & LIBIDO DURING PREGNANCY

by Dr Mpume Zenda

Hormonal changes occur during and post pregnancy. Sex drive or libido (the desire to have sex) is generally decreased in the first trimester owing to the hormonal changes, but also minor ailments of pregnancy such as nausea and vomiting and extreme tiredness make it harder to want to be intimate.

The second trimester is marked with an increased sex desire owing to increased fluid which causes more blood to be channeled to the reproductive organs for the growing baby, marked by an increase in vaginal lubrication and overall sensation. Together with the subsiding morning sickness and psychological settling into the pregnancy one can experience a sudden increase in sex drive.

In the third trimester once again, sexual function tends to decline as a result from the discomfort of being highly pregnant, fatigue and delivery anxiety. All of this is quite normal so be gentle with yourself and take all the help you can get.

Write down any difficulties in your pregnancy that you would like to process:

"The only way into the universe is through the body of a woman."

- John O'Donoghue

BIRTH OPTIONS
by Caitlin

Most women go into a birth expecting there to be two options: normal delivery or cesarean section. While on paper this might be true, in reality, there is a lot more to it. I cannot stress enough that the most important thing about a birth plan is creating a space where the mum feels safe and empowered to trust her body and the baby that her body has grown. Each mum knows herself the best and has her reasons for choosing the birth that she does. There is no 'better' birth than another. Each requires the mum to physically put herself second to the child she brings into the world, thereby offering her first sacrifice as a mum.

Most women's biggest fear around labour is how they will cope with the pain. There are a lot of different options available to help you manage the physical contractions and the anxiety that can weaken your sense of control. It is possible to labour without pain medication but you will need to put time into mental preparation. The pain is different from anything that you will have experienced before and it helps immensely to be physically and mentally strong. You are more than capable of controlling the impact the pain has, if you practise the skills that help you to channel your energy towards a calm, surrendered strength.

It is important to reframe the pain as natural and positive rather than it being a negative signal to your body (such as the pain if you were to break a bone).

> The 'fear-tension-pain' cycle describes how pain can become intensified if we fear it. Therefore, it is key to use tools (such as deep breathing, posture, affirmations, relaxing music etc.) to relax one's body and mind during contractions.

If you view the pain as having a purpose, it helps immensely. The main source of pain is due to the longitudinal and latitudinal muscles of your uterus contracting in an effort to open your cervix and push your baby down. Remember this when you experience contractions - this work is natural and has a purpose. Instead of resisting it by clenching your body, rather relax and give in to it. Pay attention to your posture and if you find yourself tensing, breathe using the technique given to you in the meditation (chapter one).

There is also no weakness in choosing to have pain medication. Some mums express disappointment that they weren't able to cope or that they 'caved in' to the pain. Those medications are there to help you to reach the end goal of a healthy birth for your baby and yourself. They assist in reducing anxiety and ease the journey. You should not feel pressured to labour in any other way than what you feel is best for yourself. This requires that you first know the options that are available to you.

Every woman that has laboured will understand that desire to reach for anything that will soften the discomfort. Your biggest ally in labour is the shy hormone oxytocin which coordinates and drives the contraction of your womb. Any feelings of anxiety or being out of control will suppress the effects of oxytocin and delay the progress to meeting your child.

Did you know?

Women in feminist movements advocated for pain relief around 1915. Hospital births became more common in the 1920s. The epidural was made available in the 1970s along with water births and hypnosis as alternatives. In the 1980s, there was a swing back to home births and birthing without pain medication. By the 2000s, a third of deliveries were done via C-section. What do you think is the discourse around birth in your culture today?

BIRTH OPTIONS

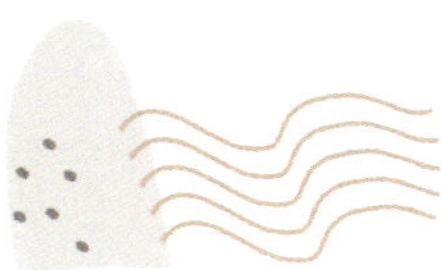

MOVEMENT AND BREATHING

Movement and breathing exercises taught at most pregnancy pilates classes are a wonderful way to physically divert your concentration to something that you can focus on and control. Mindfulness and meditation can also calm through distracting the mind. Hypnobirthing teaches specific techniques to focus thoughts and movements on relieving the discomfort of pregnancy surges.

WATER BIRTH

Many women choose to labour in a birthing pool, using the warm water to ease lower back discomfort and help hold the weight of the tummy. For some, the warmth may slow contractions so your midwife might ask you to get out the water to speed things up again or to only enter the bath in the advanced stages of labour for a water birth.

TENS MACHINE

A TENS machine is something best used in early labour to 'take the edge off' the contractions. It is a series of pads that you stick onto your lower back to deliver a small shock that triggers your brain to feel this, over the pain of labour. As the contractions increase in intensity, you can increase the strength of the impulse on your back. It works best if applied when you are at home and navigating the first, regular labour pains. You can use the TENS machine to alleviate Braxton Hicks labour pains (irregular practise contractions felt in the days or weeks before labour).

Medical pain management depends on where you choose to labour. Midwives that attend home births are often equipped with oral pain medication and some muscle injections that can both calm anxiety and help with pain. They cannot usually offer more than this and you will need to mentally prepare to cope without more effective pain medication. In a hospital setting you may have access to slightly stronger muscle injections like Pethidine, gas and air masks and an epidural. Once you know more about the various pain medications, speak to your health professional and find out what options can be made available to you. A birth plan should be flexible and lightly held depending on your and your baby's needs on the day. It is helpful to practise Hypnobirthing or meditation to navigate the early stages of labour calmly, regardless of how you are to give birth.

PETHIDINE

Pethidine is an opioid like Morphine which softens the pain and helps you to cope. Like most opioids, it can make you feel nauseous and, if given close to the time of delivery, can make your baby a bit more sleepy than usual. The birth attendants will know to look out for this and can give a light reversal agent if needed.

GAS

Gas and air is also called Entonox and is a combination of oxygen and nitrous oxide that will take the edge off the contractions. It can make you feel quite light headed and nauseous but is a game changer in the later hours of labour just before delivery. It is breathed in through a face mask and helps to co-ordinate your breathing and your remaining energy even while pushing.

EPIDURAL

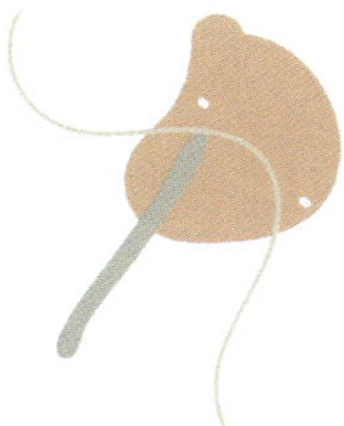

An epidural can be miraculous or a huge disappointment. It involves inserting a thin, long needle into your lower back to place a line that can give you small amounts of local anaesthetic to numb your nerves that detect pain in your lower body. You might have heard of mums that were able to rest as their labour progressed without them feeling a thing. Others will tell of being numb in one leg and feeling everything in the other. It all depends on whether the local anaesthetic bathes both sides of the spinal cord equally. The doctor will need to put in an intravenous drip and catheter and it is common for your blood pressure to drop, making you feel light headed.

They will also attach a CTG belt to your tummy to monitor your baby's heartbeat with each contraction. The need for monitoring will restrict your movement and often means that you are lying on your back in a bed and will labour in this position. When it is time to push, the doctor will turn the epidural down so that you can feel the contractions, but this too does not always work and may be the reason for an increased need for assisted deliveries using vacuum or forceps.

If you choose to have a cesarean section or your baby goes into fetal distress during labour you will be given a spinal block. This is similar to an epidural but a larger dose of local anaesthetic is given to completely numb the lower half of your body. It is normal to shiver and feel a little nauseous. The anaesthetist will monitor you and may spray a cold liquid on your chest to check the 'level' of the spinal. Sometimes a spinal may go too high and make it difficult to breathe deeply. There are times when the anaesthetist may put a face mask over your mouth and nose to give you more oxygen to improve oxygen supply to the baby. You will feel the pressure and movements of the obstetrician as they progress to get your baby out but you will not feel it as pain.

The only exception to this is if the baby is very premature or the mother is very unwell when a general anaesthetic is done. You will need to be put to sleep and your partner will not be allowed to remain in the theatre for the surgery but can go with your baby to the nursery once it is delivered.

Sometimes, before you have gone into labour naturally, you may need to be induced. This is a decision that will be made by your health carer for your safety or for that of your baby. It may be that your blood pressure has gone too high and you are getting symptoms like headaches, blurred vision or a puffy face or it may be because your placenta is no longer growing your baby and the ultrasound has shown poor blood flow or a plateau in the growth. You should not have an induction if you are well and your baby is well. It is better to allow your body to go into labour naturally, if it is safe to do so. Trust your body and your baby to know when they are ready.

An induction can take many forms:
A simple sweep of the cervix will stretch the glands at its mouth that release a chemical called prostaglandin that will stimulate oxytocin release. Sometimes they will give a pessary or gel of prostaglandins at the mouth of the cervix to have the same effect. These methods will not cause stronger labour pains as they allow the body to produce its own oxytocin, but they may require longer time to have effect, especially when the body was not ready for labour.

Oxytocin is the hormone that causes the contraction of the two layers of muscle in the uterus. This muscle contraction shortens the cervix and pulls the sides apart to allow it to dilate. It also creates a pushing force at the top of the uterus to guide the baby down through the pelvis. There are synthetic forms of oxytocin that are given as a drip into your vein that will cause uterine contractions. This can cause stronger contractions and is often only given with an epidural for pain relief.

Use this acronym in discerning what forms of pain relief you are open to in your birth plan:

B	Benefits: Why might this option be beneficial?
R	Risks: What are the risks?
A	Alternatives: What other options are available?
I	Instincts: What are your instincts telling you?
N	Nothing: What if I was to wait out the labour and choose no pain relief?

Each birth process is different and the woman going into that birth will be richer and stronger coming out. It is empowering but humbling. Allow yourself to ask for help. Listen to your body and trust it, together with your baby, to know how best to manage. And trust your birth attendants to guide you both safely through.

"It is important to keep in mind that our bodies must work pretty well, or there wouldn't be so many humans on the planet."

- Ina May Gaskin

BEING EMPOWERED

by Caitlin

Regardless of whether or not your birth goes according to plan, it is possible to be empowered in the process. The way you feel going into birth will depend on how well supported you are and the 'team' of people around you. It is vital for you to acquire relevant knowledge in those forty weeks of pregnancy so that you can make decisions that are well-informed and make you feel safe and strong.

It is important to know the pros and cons of both cesarean and natural births and to know the possibilities of what might happen to change your chosen course. Things can change quickly in labour and you may witness a 'cascade of interventions' happening around you. It is good to learn to trust your body but also to trust your carer so that, when a decision is made, you feel considered and cared for rather than medically managed.

One of the biggest decisions that you will need to make is the choice of your health carer. This might be the local Midwife Obstetric Team supervised by a consultant, a private midwife or a private Obstetrician. Spend some time reading about what their views are on birth and whether those align with yours.

Look at the statistics from their recent births and how many natural births, instrumental and cesarean deliveries they have done. You will need to bear in mind that doctors are not necessarily present unless they are needed for an intervention.

Uncomplicated deliveries are usually managed by midwives, so when viewing the doctors statistics, look at whether they support midwife lead deliveries if that is something you are hoping for.

Think about who you might like to be present when you are labouring. Some women feel best supported by a partner or mum, while others might also want the support of a doula or birthing companion. A doula is someone that can help manage both your experience, and that of your partner; facilitating movement, helpful breathing and focus. You can also discuss and decide who you would like to 'catch' the baby and whether you want to experience skin-to-skin when the baby is born. If you already have children, you will need to decide whether they will be there while you labour and who will be available to look after them.

Your birthing environment will also set the tone for your labour experience. You will need to decide if you would like to birth at home or how you feel about birthing in a hospital. Not all hospitals have access to birthing pools or birthing stools and some might place more pressure on lying on a bed. You might want to birth in a private room or might be open to labouring in a general ward and moving to a delivery room when the time comes to deliver. You will also need to make a decision about where you want to recover. Some hospitals offer private rooms where your partner can stay overnight but this is usually at an additional cost. Go for a hospital tour, even a virtual one, and ask all of these questions so that you are familiar with the environment in which you will labour. Visualise how you can make it as comfortable as you can with music, candles and dimmed lights.

Feeling empowered requires you to create a sacred space that will place you in the best position to labour. Gathering information beforehand to make those valuable decisions, with your healthcare provider, will allow you to trust your instincts and give you confidence that your health carer knows what you desire. Ultimately, you need to surrender to the process and know that things might not go according to plan but that it is possible to feel calm and in control.

CAITLIN'S STORY ON WHO WAS PRESENT AT HER SECOND LABOUR:

I remember thinking about who I wanted to be with me while I laboured and who I wanted to look after Peter. My mum is such a source of strength to me, but she had not been able to be present when Peter was born. I felt that Dave and I had shared such a growing experience during my first labour so I really wanted him to be with me again. I made the decision for my parents to have Peter for the night I went into labour and the few nights after, while I was in hospital. It was such a reassurance knowing that I could make the call whenever I went into labour and they would be there to pick up my son and love him while I was away. My husband was so much more incredible in supporting me the second time around because he recognised the difficulties from before and was far better equipped to manage them.

"Birth is vast and multifaceted; radiant and mysterious. Birth contains multitudes, and through her we birth our multitudes. We give birth to our hopes and our fears, to our ecstasies and our agonies, to our joy and our disappointments. We give birth to our babies, each one perfect and radiant. We give birth through our instincts, and we give birth to our instincts. We give birth to our capacity for instincts, which will match us perfectly with our babies, who are, and always will be, instinctive creatures. May we all be blessed through instinctive birth."

- Dr Sarah Buckley

Birth Plan

• How do you feel about labour?

• Who do you want with you while you labour?

• Who would you like to 'catch' the baby when they are born?

• What pain management would you like?

- Movement and breathing
- Meditation
- TENS machine
- Massage
- Warm water
- Pain tablets
- Injectable pain relief
- Gas and air
- Epidural

• How would you like to labour?

- In water
- In bed
- Squatting
- Standing

• Where would you like to labour?

- At home
- In hospital
- An elective Cesarean Section

• Do you (or a partner) want to do 'skin-to-skin' where the baby is held against your bare chest straight after it is born?

• If you have chosen to breastfeed, would you like help latching the baby after he/she is born?

• Where would you like to recover?

- At home
- In a general hospital ward
- In a private hospital room with a partner or close friend or family member

"It is impossible to be a perfect mother, but there are a million ways to be a good one."

- 'Proud Happy Mama' Blog

EMOTIONS AROUND BIRTH

by Charlene Yared West

Birth can be one of the most positive and empowering experiences of a woman's life, where she steps into matrescence (the transition into motherhood) leaving her old self behind. Birth does not have to be a fearful event and Hypnobirthing can help her to have a birth free from fear, no matter what kind of birth she has, or what turn it takes.

A birth free of fear is a better birth - every time! Even an abdominal birth can be an empowered one, where mom and baby connect and bond. Another word for Hypnobirthing might as well be 'Relax-o-Birthing' where the mother takes herself into a deep state of calm, relaxation and courage to help herself through labour.

When a mother is reminded of her innate power to birth her baby using Hypnobirthing, it has far reaching effects into her postpartum and motherhood journey.

Hypnobirthing gives her a toolkit of natural pain relief and relaxation techniques that she can use on the day she gives birth and beyond, which includes: evidence based birthing information, positive affirmations, mindfulness techniques, visualizations, massage, aromatherapy, birth environment tips and tricks, as well as training for her birth partner. These topics are included in the Relax Into Birth Hypnobirthing online course.

My aim at every birth is to mirror exactly what the mother needs in any given situation, so that the experience she has is a positive one. My experience has taught me how important it is to educate and support mothers through their pregnancy, labour and birth so that they know they have options available to them to make informed decisions at every point on their birthing journey.

Each mother has a birth story to share – may her journey to birth and beyond be an empowered one.

www.learn-hypnobirthing.relaxintobirth.com

www.relaxintobirth.com/homestudy-online-hypnobirthing-course

PREGNANCY IN GRIEF

by Caitlin

Pregnancy after loss is full of a range of feelings and all of them are valid. While many women experience miscarriages, ectopic pregnancy, abnormalities on ultrasound scans or infant death, little space is allowed for you to process those feelings. It is sometimes hard to know when it is appropriate to talk about this. It is difficult to know how much to say. Many women internalise the emotions they have for fear of making others feel uncomfortable.

This can become a problem when you discover that you are pregnant again. As much as you want to hope for the best, fear that the same thing will happen in this pregnancy can drown out any joy. It is okay for you to guard your emotions or to even feel guilt for the child that you have lost. It is okay to be on the journey through grief, as it is likely to be a journey that you will be on forever. Any child conceived, is a child that has lived and a child that will be loved forever.

People might tell you to 'be positive' or to 'hope for the best'. It is normal to resent comments like this and to feel angry about not being able to be joyful about your pregnancy. Find a safe space to be honest about your feelings and set boundaries on conversations or comments that you don't feel comfortable with. Close those conversations off by saying 'thank you' and carry that discomfort to your safe space by writing them down or talking them through with your safe person.

Allow yourself the space to feel your grief and your joy. This pregnancy will not steal from a previous pregnancy. Try to accept your anger and even the blame you have allocated, before your child is born, so that you can freely celebrate this new life. Each pregnancy is unique and it is safe to look on each one with the experience and perspectives you have gained.

Know that your partner will be mourning in their own way. Some might share your feelings but some might grieve in a different way. Allow them to process the experience in the way that they feel comfortable but always reinforce that they are loved and that it is safe for them to be honest about whatever they may feel. Try not to take on their emotion but rather act as a sounding board to help them understand what they feel. It can be difficult to reach this balance as we naturally hear blame where it may not have been intended.

Although it might feel like the hardest thing to do, try to speak to close friends and family. Finding out that someone has gone through something similar and having a safe space to name what you feel as alright, helps to gain control. Be gentle and take each day, each moment; one step at a time.

PREPARING TO TAKE CARE OF YOUR BODY

by Caitlin

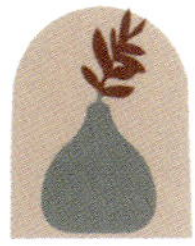

The days after delivery can be a bit of a blur. You have climbed the mountain and reached your reward and yet find yourself standing before the unknown. While millions of women have faced this before, we have greatly underappreciated the gravity of what our bodies have done, and what is expected of mothers in the days and weeks ahead. It is most important for you to know that you will have days when you feel tired, confused, resentful, sore and alone. Similarly you will feel gratitude, relief and immeasurable joy. And some days you might feel it all. It helps to be gentle with yourself and to put things in place that will help to ease the load of demands in the first few weeks at home.

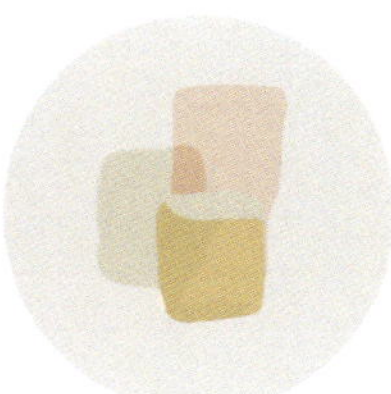

POST DELIVERY

Depending on what sort of labour you have had you will find little physical comforts that can ease the pain and speed up recovery.

A pelvic ice pack is a great way to soothe the pain of vaginal tears or an episiotomy. Alternatively, make your own 'padsicles' by applying Aloe Vera gel and/or lavender essential oil and witch hazel to pads which you can then freeze and wear as a normal pad to ease swelling.

A doughnut pillow might be helpful if you experience discomfort when sitting.

SITZ BATHS

Add coarse salt to a small bowl of warm water and soak in it twice a day to prevent infection if you've had a vaginal tear or an episiotomy. Allow the area to air and even use a hairdryer to dry the area before putting on your underwear.

A 'peri-spray' can be used to spray the perineum after you use the bathroom. Buy a spray bottle and add coarse salt to warm water.

PAIN MANAGEMENT

Take pain medication to help you get up and move as you will need to pick up, feed and bath your baby. Once your wounds have closed you can begin to massage natural oils (like coconut oil) into the scars to soften and assist with healing.

NIPPLE CARE

Purchase a baby friendly nipple cream (such as Lansinoh) that you can apply before and after feeds. This can soothe cracked nipples and the sandpaper feeling of your baby's tongue. You can also massage breastmilk into the areola after feeding. Let your nipples air and even better, give them some time in the sun. Certain women's health physiotherapists can offer laser therapy to treat cracked, sore nipples.

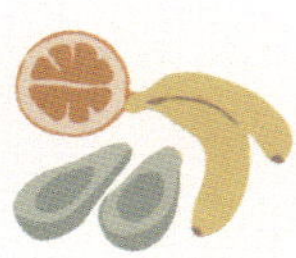

NUTRITION

In order for your body to recover and to make the nutrient rich breast milk to nourish your baby, you will need to feed and nourish yourself. Continue to take your antenatal supplements and consider taking extra zinc, vitamin C and iron to boost soft tissue repair and replace what was lost through labour. Stock up on quick snacks like oat breakfast bars and energy bars.

Spend a few days, ahead of your due date, making dinners that can be frozen or ask a reliable family member or close friend to organize a roster of people to make dinners for you in the first week at home with your newborn.

YOUR HOME

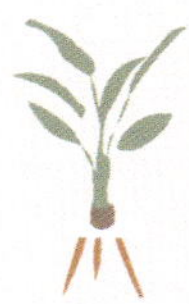

Try to set up your home to be as supportive as possible. Put together a basket with some nappies, wipes and a changing mat that you can use in the lounge as well as one in your baby changing area. Have some muslin burping cloths and a few change of clothes in the basket too. Invest in a dimmed light that you can easily reach when you wake in the middle of the night to feed. Keep your slippers and a gown or blanket nearby for those colder nights that you need to keep yourself warm.

BODY IMAGE

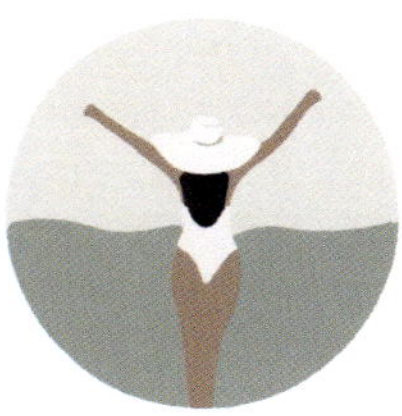

The first few weeks after having a baby are the most difficult in terms of your physical body. Your womb takes time to shrink back to its original size of a fist and you can carry a residual tummy that takes a little longer to disappear than you may have hoped. Don't forget that you have grown and birthed a human being and that you may not simply 'get back to normal'. Wear those physical scars with pride at the knowledge of what you have achieved. Don't try to exercise your core too soon as it may restrict your abdominal muscles from coming back together, resulting in a gap called diastasis recti and even an umbilical hernia. It will also interfere with your skin knitting back together, causing poor wound healing of cesarean and vaginal scars. Movement is good as long as you listen to your body and stop when you feel things pulling or causing pain. You can wear an abdominal support band to help hold the skin and muscles together. Wear dark trousers to hide blood stains from the lochia that slowly clears the blood from your womb and wear lighter tops to hide milk spills. It helps to wear a double layer while breastfeeding so that the inner top can be moved down and the outer top can be moved up creating a dignified 'window' to access your nipple. In hot weather, wearing button down shirts and dresses is helpful.

REDEFINING SUCCESS AS A MOTHER

by Caryn

I remember feeling particularly triggered when Sienna was a newborn and someone asked me if she was a 'good' baby. What did they mean by 'good'? As far as I was concerned, babies couldn't be 'bad'. This common question seems to refer to: "Is she a content baby? Does she not cry, does she just sit happily gurgling to herself?" No, this was not the case for me, and I felt annoyed that I was even asked this question. Babies communicate through crying. Babies like to be held and engaged because they are wired for connection. All babies have needs and some are more outspoken than others - this does not make them bad and it does not make me a bad mother.

I have realised while navigating the challenge of discipline with my toddler that I tend to internalise her behaviour - that sometimes I take her reactions as a reflection of my parenting rather than allowing space for her learning. I have learnt to see it as developmentally appropriate for some level of 'push back' and view it as a learning curve objectively and independent of me. It has made me realise how easy it is to slip into guilt and shame as a mother in various stages of parenting. Let's talk about the difference in their essence:

Guilt is feeling bad about what I've done. Shame is feeling bad about who I am.

Guilt is a helpful emotion insofar as it signals to me an area of improvement. If I allow it to paralyse me, however, it becomes unhelpful. If I can become curious about it, view it from a distance, emotionally separating it from my world for a moment and allow it to become my teacher, then there is an opportunity for transformation. Perhaps I feel guilty about not connecting properly with my child, then I can think about some shifts I can make to be more intentional about communicating with her. Do you see that this is the value guilt can offer as long as it doesn't swallow you up? Here in this area, I can see that I can do a better job, and even in this, I can still talk kindly to myself. I'm trying my best... sometimes I fail... and that's okay because I'm willing to learn and try again.

Shame goes deeper. It signals a feeling of unworthiness. It brings up self-loathing. If I want to heal from this, I can still navigate it by becoming curious, to ask why it might be my experience, but it usually signals that I might need some support to find healing.

Inevitably, you will feel that you fail at something along the way. You might be wrestling with your stance versus the myriad of parenting opinions. You might feel guilt about juggling work and motherhood or desire some time away from your children. You might feel guilt about not being able to breastfeed - or for as long as you had hoped. You could feel guilty for not always enjoying being a mother. In these times, pay attention to when guilt becomes shame - when guilt makes you feel like you're not a good mother. Defining your 'good enough' is imperative in this battle.

We've discussed the myth of a good baby. You might find yourself questioning whether you are a good mother at times - and if you hold yourself to an unrealistic standard or battle to accept difficult emotions, this can lead to shame. Here is a tool to help you navigate this:

What are your values as a mother?

- Name the qualities that you already possess which will make you a good mother in your unique way.
- Name and describe some traits and actions that you feel constitute good parenting.
- Without the intention of comparing yourself to another, name some of the qualities you admire in mothers who have inspired you.
- What do you think is the standard of success for mothers in your family, peer group and society?

Let this be a chance for you to think critically about whether or not you agree with this (such as, a good Mom is keen to explore homeschooling or a successful Mom is able to find the correct balance between the demands of work and home).

A good mother doesn't equate to 'perfect'. A good mother measures her success against her own values rather than the expectations of others. She might not meet these standards at times, but she is a good mother because she continually returns to what she hopes to be. In this way, she parents with integrity rather than the impossible feat of perfection. Integrity is aligning herself to her own standard of success when she feels she's missing the mark. She can lie in bed at night and know she has done a good job not because it was perfect, but because she is willing to improve. You aren't perfect, but you are good enough.

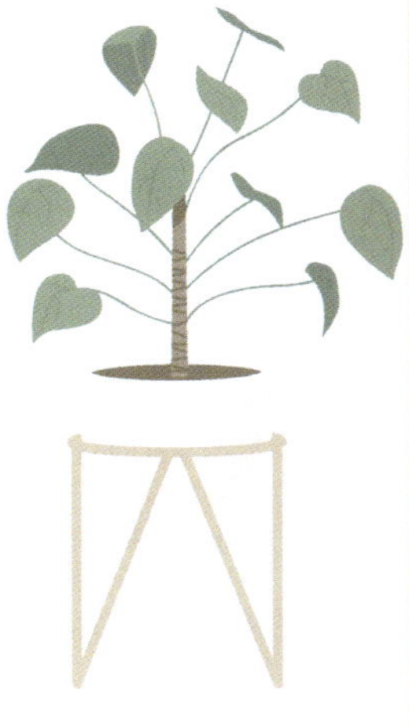

MAMA'S VALUES

A good mother measures her success against her own values rather than the expectations of others.

What is *your* 'good enough'?

- Reflect once again on your values. Summarise them according to who you are and who you hope to be, being realistic about how you perceive success.
- Summarise this into five points which you aim to live by in your relationship with your child.

These ideas will continue to form over time. These developing values will be your metric of success. They are an anchor when you feel you're flailing in guilt and perfectionism.

Return to this set of values often as a way to guide you back to integrity rather than steering you towards guilt and shame. Perhaps print it out and stick it up in a place where you'll see it often.

EXPECTATIONS FOR THE FOURTH TRIMESTER

by Caryn

It is impossible to be totally prepared for motherhood. While motherhood is an incredible privilege, it's okay to acknowledge that postpartum is a raw and fragile time of navigating your own healing and identity shift while sustaining a little life completely dependent on you. You do not have to enjoy every minute of motherhood in order to be a good mother! When have you ever been expected to feel grateful all of the time? It's no different for motherhood; and exhibiting uncomfortable emotions on some days and during various seasons of life, doesn't mean you don't love your child.

Perhaps you have never heard of the fourth trimester, and you are nearing the end of your pregnancy and counting down the days to feel like you have your body back and to be freed from the discomfort. Consider, however, that there is another trimester to go - and give yourself permission to rest and be patient with the connection being forged between you and your baby as you 'learn' each other.

The first three months of your baby's life is known as the 'fourth trimester' for the very reason that human babies would do well to endure a final trimester in utero - only, they would be too big to birth. Think of all other mammals - they are almost able to stand and fend for themselves from their day of birth. Human babies, on the other hand, need their every need met by their mothers... and in many ways, still think they are in the womb. This is illustrated by the five 'S' words that you can practise in the fourth trimester:

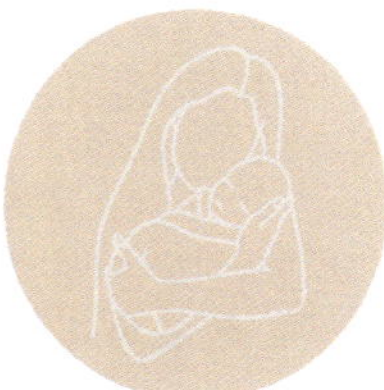

SWADDLE

Babies are used to being held tightly in the womb. Often their flailing arms wake them up. Swaddling babies tightly to calm them or help them sleep might be useful. Don't be alarmed if your baby resists it, but perhaps give it a try. Swaddling is not recommended during breastfeeding as allowing their hands to roam is important for their development.

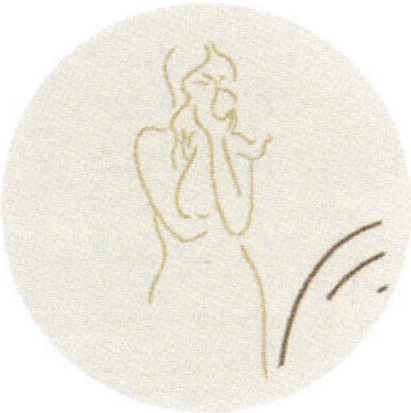

SWAY

Your baby is accustomed to the movement of being in utero. This is why babies generally fall asleep easily when in the car, pram or being worn in a carrier. Swaying comes naturally to a mum trying to soothe her baby. When your baby is fussy or needs to sleep, draw on movement as a tool and don't be worried if the cot is standing dormant for many of the naps in these early days.

SUCK

Babies do not only breastfeed for nutrition, but for comfort too. You might have a baby who will fuss and fuss until he or she is able to suck on something. Some babies will suck on your breast, even if they are full, for comfort as they fall asleep. Some take dummies and others refuse them.Dummies are the preferential option to thumb-sucking as they can be gently phased out when the time comes for your child to learn other means of comfort.

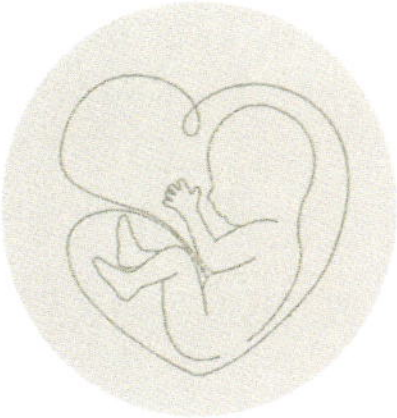

SHUSH

The womb is noisy! Your baby might prefer white noise which mimics sounds in the womb than sleeping in a dead quiet room. There are sound machines and apps available which can help your baby form a sleep association to the comforting sound of white noise. Be aware that you may need to keep the white noise throughout the night as they will listen for it when they wake in the night as the association to go back to sleep. It is also recommended that you allow for some natural noise to be present during naps in the day so that they can differentiate between day and night.

SKIN-TO-SKIN

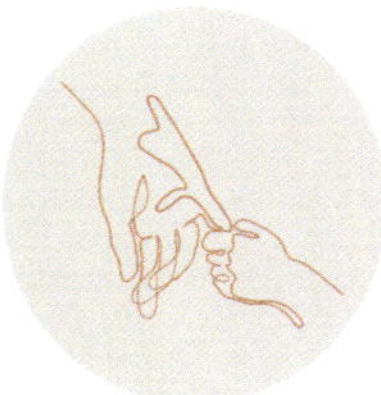

Babies love to be close to their caregivers and to hear their beating heart as when they were in utero. Whether your baby is breastfeeding or taking a bottle, skin-to-skin helps nurture a stronger connection and has physiological benefits such as: increasing milk let down and contraction of the uterus due to the hormone oxytocin and decreasing baby's blood pressure and helping them settle through secure attachment. It is common for mums to find that their babies only want to sleep on them. If you are finding this demanding, try wearing your baby in a sling or carrier. Persist with it even if your baby doesn't enjoy getting into it in the beginning - they may get used to it and can have lovely long sleeps when safely worn. Make sure that their airway is visible, that their head is 'close enough to kiss' and that they are not overdressed as they can't regulate their own body temperature.

Despite how cute your tiny newborn will be and how you might feel overcome by loving emotions at times, it is expected that there will be a feeling of overwhelm for part or much of the fourth trimester. There is perhaps no other task in life as intensive as caring for a newborn. Babies are so cute to ensure that we secure an attachment with them, making the hard days of caring for them easier because of those chubby cheeks and button nose!

Be honest about your feelings. Know that it is okay if you feel depleted emotionally and physically, but be sure to reach out for the support that you need. This is where you can turn to the knowledge of what moods and emotions can be expected; and those which might be signposting a flag for specialised support. You can also use the self-coaching session where you will learn how to draw on a support system and implement a postpartum care plan.

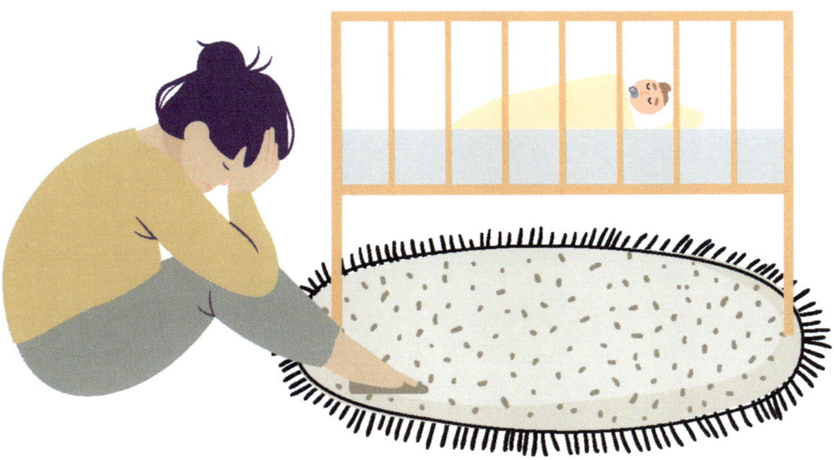

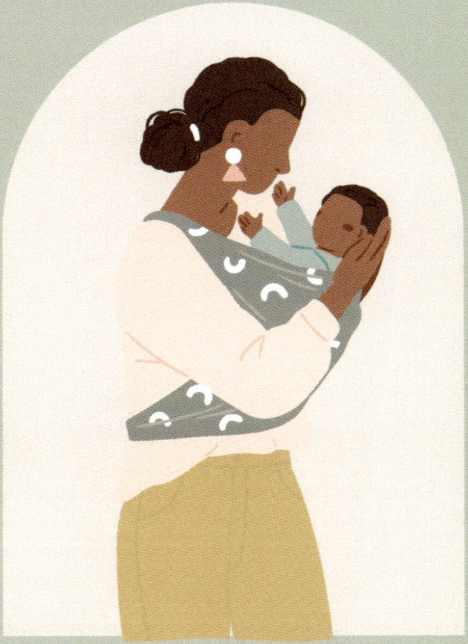

Holding Mama

A POST PARTUM SUPPORT PLAN

by Caryn

This chapter is designed to help you identify ways to support yourself through what we have named the Four 'Rs' of rest, refill, rhythm and requests.

Essentially, by finding ways to hold yourself and requesting ways that others can hold you is an act of self-care. In generations past, mothers tended to become martyrs to the needs of the family and, in turn, neglect their own well-being. Perhaps the focus on self-care can be perceived as selfish as motherhood is a path of intense giving. We would like to help you see that self-care is selfless: a mum cannot pour from an empty cup. She needs to rest, refill and connect with others. She needs to express her needs and make requests for support. It fascinates us that there are often so many tangible signs of support when a woman is pregnant - she is encouraged to put her feet up, she is asked how she is feeling, she is showered with gifts for the baby - yet when the baby arrives, the community often seems to have gone silent. Perhaps some meals are provided and people hold the baby, but where is the village to hold mum? Do friends text to ask how they can support her or does conversation revolve mainly around the new baby? In finding ways to hold herself and by allowing others to hold her, she can hold the baby with arms that are at greater ease, outstretched to give again.

THE FOUR R's - REST, REFILL, RHYTHM & REQUESTS

by Caryn

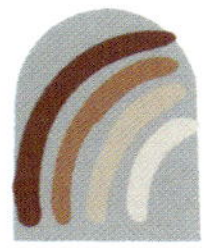

For new mums, some days can just feel monotonous. For some it can be lonely if you find it hard to reach adult conversation or if you live far from family. When I had Sienna, it felt like my day was divided into feeding slots and I would count how many naps she had and, more pressingly, the hours until my husband would be home and I could sneak in a glass of wine after a feed. So how does one find meaning in a day revolving from one nappy change to the next? Or for moms with busy schedules or multiple kids - how does one even find the time?

There are FIVE experiences to seek out in a day in order to find rhythm. This will break the monotony and add grounding when it feels like you're just giving, giving, giving.

Five things to do each day to keep your soul in check:

RITUAL	**Wake up right** Replace checking your phone as you awake, with a morning ritual such as prayer/meditation/deep breathing/a stretch/a gratitude list/lighting a candle.
HOPES	**While a to-do list is great, it can feel like pressure to get all the things done** Rather focus on 1-3 things that you'll be happy you did/experienced by the end of the day. More than 'to-do', focus on building in hopes so that you can also focus on 'being' rather than just doing.
CONNECT	**Be intentionally present** For at least ten minutes, aim to give deliberate attention to someone in your family (no phones/tasks/distractions). Alternatively, or in addition, you can message or serve someone in some way.

MOVE	**Get moving** Get moving for 20 minutes without the goal of fitness or weight loss. Simply think of it as getting your blood flowing, body stretching and heart beating. Maybe it's a walk or stretch, cardio session or tidy around the house.
REFLECT	**Take 5 minutes to notice the day that has passed:** What brought you connection and joy? What brought disconnection and lack of joy? What does this tell you about what you can do to move forward into tomorrow?

If you start building in these things intentionally, they'll eventually become habits that then give a rhythm to your day. Don't get hung up if you don't do them all, but notice how you start to crave the variety and feeling of being grounded that they provide. And if you battle to do them all, start with one and build it up.

BUT, the key is to have low expectations and give yourself lots of grace if you don't manage to do them all. It's more of a compass in times of depletion, giving you direction to feel on course again.

With Sienna, I spent a lot of our nursing sessions watching Netflix. With Kolbe, I am more intentional about feeding my soul in other ways and I'm also more accepting that as an introvert, I will have company 24/7. But knowing how quickly time goes (although it may not feel like it at the time), I have the perspective that just as their routine changes, so will mine. Find time for things in the ebb and flow.

If I seek out these experiences, I am more likely to feel refilled and less likely to count the hours. Being flexible as to when and how long I can do these things is also key. Sometimes we need to 'fight' for the time and make it a priority when life is busy. This could mean asking one's partner to step in (which is sometimes not easy nor simple as there can be a lot of tension around finding time for oneself especially if one partner feels that the 'load' is unequal). This is why the art of making REQUESTS is so important; an obvious yet difficult skill at times. I coach my clients on this very point.

Lastly, communicating to those around you and making a request of someone (e.g. a partner) to help you implement this might be necessary — such as allowing you 20 minutes of space to wake up right, formulate your hopes for the day, connect, move or reflect. It's also about being flexible and allowing it to look different each day. For me, all of this includes having a newborn at my side; and usually a toddler too!

> **"The most difficult part of birth is the first year afterwards. It is the year of travail – when the soul of a woman must birth the mother inside her. The emotional labour pains of becoming a mother are far greater than the physical pangs of birth; these are the growing surges of your heart as it pushes out selfishness and fear and makes room for sacrifice and love. It is a private and silent birth of the soul, but it is no less holy than the event of childbirth, perhaps it is even more sacred."**
>
> *- Joy Kusek*

What existing practices do you use to keep your soul in check?

See how your week progresses and take your energy levels and mental wellness as an indication of when and how you can change pace and bring in some varied experiences such as a walk, coffee date or nap. Perhaps earmark Friday as a slower day where you give yourself permission to rest or refill (the difference between these terms is discussed later on in the book) especially if you're feeling like it's been a tough week.

REFILL

Below are some questions to help you consider what refills you. By incorporating these things you will hopefully find rhythm to ground you, as you embrace your new way of being as a mother.

WHAT/WHO REFILLS ME IN GIVING ME?

e.g. running/friendships

EXPLANATION	HOW I REFILL
JOY (inspiration, excitement, purpose etc.)	
PEACE (feeling grounded, calm, capable)	
CONNECTION (Activities and relationships that make me feel connected to myself and others). Mention particular relationships where you would like to nurture connection.	

RHYTHM

Choose ONE activity/relationship from the categories (joy, peace and connection) which you can incorporate weekly. Explain how you might do this and, if it is relevant, what request might need to be made in order to make this happen. By aiming to do at least one of these things each week, a rhythm will be established and you will start to find integration in your new way of life.

WHAT	HOW	WHO
JOY		
PEACE		
CONNECTION		

SUPPORT

It is vital to seek support by making requests respectfully and assertively.

WHO CAN SUPPORT ME IN THESE AREAS IF I EVER NEED HELP?

WHAT?	WHO?
DAY-TO-DAY (groceries/errands before or after baby's birth	
MEALS (drawing up a meal roster)	
EMOTIONAL WELLBEING (someone I can be vulnerable with)	
OTHER (any other areas I need help now or in the future)	

MAKING REQUESTS

Some of us are more used to making requests than others. It can be challenging to ask for what we need because many of us don't want to seem demanding. Reflect on how you make requests - are you assertive, too demanding, submissive or do you avoid making requests at all costs so as not to inconvenience anyone?

USE THIS SPACE TO JOURNAL

Write down what language you use when requesting something:

What emotions do you feel when making a request?

Write down what body language you use. You might be communicating your mood non-verbally which makes the recipient react in a certain way.

You cannot pour from an empty cup so perhaps you need to reframe how you make requests - it is not a selfish act to ask for help. Can someone hold your baby for 20 minutes while you wash your hair? Can someone pop in for a chat because you desire adult conversation? Can someone go to the store to buy you more maternity pads? There are so many kinds of needs in the early weeks of rearing a baby and making a simple request can shift your mood from overwhelm and anxiety to the wonder of having support, knowing that it's one less thing to worry about.

Practise making a request by making sure it ticks these three boxes in your language, mood and body:

- Are you clear about what you are asking?
- Is it assertive rather than apologetic?
- Is it respectful rather than demanding?

Make time to have a conversations with your partner about the following points:

What will help us, as individuals, to refill?

When can we make time for each other to do the activity of our choice? *(Perhaps it is as short as an hour per week in the early days of having a baby, but even this can help both of you).*

When you are feeling triggered by not having enough rest or refill, how do you interact with me and others?

When you notice your partner is triggered because you can identify the behaviour they describe in this question, this will become a red flag for recognising that they might need rest and refill. It is important to notice it within yourself too. Perhaps you can be more generous with the other person in giving them some time to tend to themselves in periods of burnout. Sometimes giving yourself or your partner that gift can bring you and your relationship back into an 'upward cycle' where the relationship takes on a more positive, hopeful tone, giving rise to more connection - rather than a 'downward cycle' of resentment and frustration.

Your Personal

POST PARTUM SUPPORT PLAN

I make time to refill by

I give my partner the time to refill by

When my days feel monotonous, I add rhythm by

As a family we create a weekly rhythm by

I respectfully make requests by advocating for what I need with a… *(describe tone of voice)* and... *(describe body language)*

When I need to honestly share my feelings *(especially if I'm not okay)* I connect with… *(name person/s)*

"Everyone says marriage should be 50/50; it's the biggest cock of bull sh! I've never heard it's never 50/50 - ever...**
Marriage is not something that's 50/50, a partnership works when you can carry their 20 or they can carry your 20."

- Brené Brown

CHANGING ROLE, A CHANGING IDENTITY.

by Caryn

One of the biggest shifts of becoming a parent is what feels like a change in identity. Perhaps it is healthier to speak about the changing role rather than identity, otherwise one's identity becomes fragile - swayed by the events of life rather than being grounded in who one is and will always be, regardless of outward happenings. However, there is arguably an inward change when becoming a mother: the goals of one's life are re-orientated to caring for children and one can perceive oneself from a different perspective.

How would I get through the uncertainty of the day? Would I get to rest and refill? I felt like I had lost my freedoms - mostly, my freedom to control things (you will soon learn that it's not easy to control a baby's routine so you might feel out of control of your own routine too). I wondered when I would find joy and integration again. It felt like I was mourning my 'old self' and my 'old life' and if I was honest, I felt in many ways that, I preferred it to this new life.

I can look back now from a place of wholeness and freedom, but it took at least two years for me to get to this place of accepting my new role. I am more accommodating of tiredness and demands made of me. I am more able to find joy in responsibilities that I had once perceived as overwhelming and burdensome. Just as I write about motherhood as a muscle that builds fitness and perseverance, so integration and joy has been found in being patient with myself as I learn this new role. This being said, patience is needed in finding one's way back to oneself in the simple actions of doing things that refill one's energy tank and ability to give; as well as finding rhythm which breaks the monotony of the days of early childhood rearing where it can feel like everything revolves around sustaining a little life (a privilege and a massive responsibility!). If moms can find rhythm in their week, they will find more meaning and fulfilment in life.

'When a baby is born, a mother is born.'

REFLECTIONS ON MY ROLES AND IDENTITY IN THE 4th TRIMESTER

by Caitlin

I remember distinctly feeling quite lost in the mundane and that there was quite a lot of guilt around that. I loved my time with Peter, I loved being at home with him and just adored him but that time was filled with all of the hardships of the unknown. When I describe my identity, who I believe myself to be, so much of that is my work. So much of my identity I place in my work. My heart is so filled with what I do and the interactions that I have with my patients. I found that my identity was lost in the mundane, and especially at night when I was alone and Peter was difficult to settle. I felt like I wasn't achieving very much. It can feel so raw and so tribal; having to just physically care for somebody. I missed my sense of productivity and my ability to effect changes in other people's lives. I'm used to being the carer with the emotional space and time for people and I just wanted to get back to that. I wasn't good at requesting help either.

A part of me mourned that I was not able to fill that role that I found most productive and that I was happiest and content in. I felt guilty for wanting that and for not relishing every moment with my child. I looked forward to going back to what I was good at and what made me feel like I had accomplished something at the end of the day.

While it is important to recognise that one's identity does not stem from what one does, it is equally important to notice that often it feels like it does. If a mother is only concerned about the wellbeing of her family at the expense of her own (for example, she no longer has hobbies or makes an effort with friends), she can feel like she has lost a sense of herself.

When I became a mum, I felt like my identity was being realigned and this was painful and challenging. Everything that had once represented freedom and enjoyment for me now looked different. I couldn't hop in the car and go somewhere when I wanted, my time was not my own, changing nappies could feel monotonous, I had to pack away outfits that weren't suitable for breastfeeding... the list continues. I would wake up every day of the fourth trimester feeling a heaviness in my heart: Would my baby nap?

JOURNAL | ROLES AND IDENTITY

Identity is a slippery word as it might be difficult for you to work out how you define yourself. Write down a couple of words or phrases to try get to the heart of who you are and how you see yourself.

Name some experiences that help you feel grounded in who you are and your capabilities.

Name the roles that you occupy currently and how these might speak to your identity and how you see yourself.

How might the transition into motherhood possibly create conflict with what grounds you; and in how you perceive yourself? e.g. If unbroken sleep is important for your well-being and mood, articulate how this might be a challenge for you. If you derive satisfaction from your job or have a need for introspective time, notice how this transition into motherhood might spark discomfort in juggling your needs and responsibilities.

On the other hand, how might this transition strengthen your identity by providing opportunities for your growth?

COMMUNICATION

by Caryn

Before approaching this topic, let's talk about the basics of communication that seem simple, but can be difficult to implement.

"I" STATEMENTS

This is perhaps the golden rule of all communication. By stating all feelings, grievances and points of conflict using this simple formula, you can avoid the rabbit hole of defensiveness and escalating conflict.

In essence, it is "I feel". Rather than pointing fingers by saying "you always" or "you never", it is humbly taking ownership of your feelings. Even if you have been wronged, it is choosing not to create a climate of defensiveness which can easily cause your partner to shut down. It is also being vulnerable by exposing what is really going on. Perhaps deeper reflection needs to happen prior to going into the conversation, as it is important that you know how you feel underneath whatever it is that is triggering you. Your partner is much more likely to respond to you lovingly and constructively if you can calmly communicate how you feel.

SIGNPOSTING THE CONVERSATION

While you might have the best intentions to resolve a conflict and want to resolve it now, the context for the conversation is important. If you or your partner are tired or it's been an intense day, perhaps schedule in some light-heartedness before broaching the subject.

Diving into the topic might not be the best idea as it could make your partner feel caught off guard. This is where signposting comes in.

NAME the feeling:
e.g. "Something is upsetting me."

Ask WHEN it can be discussed:
"And I would like to chat with you when you feel ready."

Take heart that "I Statements" and signposting are such simple tools. They're not always easy to implement and they don't guarantee that they will be well-received every single time, but by using them you are guaranteed to know that you've tried your best to create a healthy setting for resolving conflict.

COMMUNICATING YOUR NEEDS AS A COUPLE

YOUR NEEDS AS A COUPLE

What will be vital to your health as a mother will be advocating for your needs. The same can be said for your partner. It is important to dialogue about what both of you need in order to refill. When one or both of you are not taken care of, it can have ripple effects on your relationship and family, becoming a source of conflict. Be aware of each other's triggers by noticing when they come up. Find ways to serve each other by advocating for both of you to have time to refill.

When we have not had time to rest and refill, we can feel easily triggered or burnt out. This can escalate conflict with your partner especially if you are unaware of what is causing the emotional dysregulation. It can also make it more difficult for you to connect with each other. As much as you might feel your need for a break is more important because you might be spending more time with your baby, it is equally important to acknowledge your partner's needs as navigating the shift of bringing in a new life has an impact on both of your emotional wellbeing.

CONFLICT & COMMUNICATION

When you have the time, it might be useful to look through the following two resources *'The Four Horsemen'* and *'Emotional Flooding'* from the Gottman Institute with your partner.

EMOTIONAL FLOODING
You might find it useful to do this survey together as a couple to better understand what triggers cause arguments to escalate.

Practise adopting healthier ways of communication through your language, mood and body in the months before your baby arrives so that new habits can be put in place. Remember to go gently on yourselves and each other in this big life shift. How can you give grace when you are both tired? What can be compromised in favour of the wellbeing of everyone? Perhaps it's okay to have an untidy house at times... perhaps it's okay to get ready made meals in the early days. It's important to request what you need within the household, but it's also important to give some slack from time to time while both of you adjust.

There will be days when you need to carry the extra load or your partner needs to carry it for you... You can do this by checking in with them and asking where they are at and then explaining your side and what you need.

THE FOUR HORSEMEN

This refers to four common behaviours (criticism, contempt, defensiveness and stonewalling) adopted by couples which end up escalating conflict. Read through and observe which ones apply to you and consider the consequences of alternative behaviour.

Criticism

This is a verbal attack on both a subtle and not so subtle level. Instead of pointing fingers, use 'I statements' and adopt a respectful tone.

Contempt

Lingering feelings of resentment create a tone of hostility in a relationship. Try not to bottle negative experiences. Resolve conflicts when they are still fresh and allow yourselves to believe in the goodness of each other, to move on by actively letting go of past hurts. Let 'I forgive you' be something you truly mean.

Defensiveness

By taking things personally or refusing to take ownership for the part you play in a conflict, the conversation will reach a dead-end. It takes humility to truly listen to what your partner is saying - even if they are not 'innocent'. By saying "tell me more" instead of "but", you are more likely to reach a peaceful resolution. You can focus on taking turns to be heard, both reflecting back what you hear the other person saying, and asking if what you have heard is accurate.

Stonewalling

When you are feeling emotionally flooded, you can shut down and be unable to communicate effectively. To counteract this, you can respectfully ask for time-out and self-soothe (give yourself compassion for the emotions you are feeling, do something to bring comfort whether it's having a cup of tea, a breath of fresh air) and return to the conversation when you are feeling more grounded.

COMMUNICATING ROLES & RESPONSIBILITIES

For many couples, the sharing of household responsibilities can be a point of contention. Add a baby to this and you might both feel overwhelmed by the additional tasks involved such as finding time to grocery shop, cook, clean. Added to this is the lack of sleep which can put both of you on edge.

Be mindful of what triggers you in your current experience of this topic and anticipate doing some work together as a couple - particularly on how you communicate in times of conflict and what roles you see yourselves playing in parenting and managing the household. It will be useful to check in from time to time, after baby arrives, so that you can avoid living in resentment if you feel the division of responsibilities is unequal. However, bear in mind the quote from Brene Brown: it's unrealistic to expect the load to be equal at all times. As a mother, you might need to make peace with doing more for the baby especially in the beginning. Your partner might be able to help you in other ways - assisting you with the shopping or giving you a chance to nap if you had a sleepless night. This is where making requests will come in handy.

COMMUNICATION | JOURNALLING

What words or phrases would you use to define your role as a mother? And the role of your partner? Jot down what immediately comes to mind as well as any aspirations and hopes.

Both of you come from a unique family background. Reflect on what you appreciate about the family values and how roles and responsibilities were shared; and what you wish to do differently as you start your own family.

Division of home responsibilities:
How will you negotiate who does what in running the household and caring for a child? Will you continue your current roles or will you share them differently to accommodate the additional demands of being a parent?

Do you feel able to talk about the division of home responsibilities? Would you prefer discussing them as they come up in parenthood or are there specific choices you'd like to make now to ensure that you both know where you stand on chores and childcare? If so, note your suggestions down here.

PATIENCE APPROACHING YOUR DUE DATE

by Caryn

At the end of your pregnancy you might be feeling frustrated by how tired and achy you feel. You will be anticipating meeting your new baby and wanting the waiting to end so that you finally hold your little love.

What you might find even more challenging are the constant comments and questions from others: "Wow, you're about to pop!" and, if they know your due date, they might inadvertently be putting pressure on you by excitedly counting down the days until baby is expected to arrive.

But due dates are seldom hit on target. Due dates are an estimate and as long as your baby is moving and you are healthy (both assessed by your care provider), your baby might be overdue for a good reason.

What can be frustrating is that during the final trimester you might start with niggles (will be discussed later on) which might signal clues that labour is imminent when, in fact, it might simply be your body preparing for the big day. This is not to say you need to dismiss any concerns about labour starting, especially if it is before you are full-term (38-40 weeks) and you certainly need to discuss these concerns with your care provider.

Adopt a 'better safe than sorry' approach even if you feel like you're asking silly questions. It is your baby and your instincts to protect him or her, that trumps any fear of what your care provider might think of you for asking.

If you are hoping for a natural delivery and are starting to become impatient around your due date, continue to rest in the knowledge that both your body and baby need to be ready for labour. There is so much pressure nowadays to get labour going when in fact, well meaning suggestions like 'walking the baby out' or scrubbing the floors or eating curry can cause more anxiety than anything else. Trust in the wisdom of your body. You do not need to know when the baby will be here. By asking for clues on how dilated your cervix is, you might become despondent if it's not the result you hope for.

Process your emotions and possible feelings of impatience and need to control the uncertainty of labour. Remember that it is normal to be impatient and to wish away the last days of pregnancy. But try to focus on what memories you can create while you wait. Go on dates, do a craft, pamper yourself and enjoy some naps!

PREPARING A SIBLING

by Caitlin

SOME WORDS BY GUEST CONTRIBUTOR HOLLY PERETZ: *PEDIATRIC OCCUPATIONAL THERAPIST*

There is no denying that bringing home a new baby is a huge life experience and transition for an older sibling. A simple way that you can ease them into this is by explaining what will happen beforehand. "New baby" type storybooks can be really helpful in this, as well as letting your older child be part of preparing baby clothes or the baby room.

At that eventful first meeting consider having a gift for the older sibling "from the baby". Some find it helpful to gift a baby doll so that the older sibling can feel part of the nurturing process. However, the greatest gift you can give to an older sibling is time - your undivided attention - whether it be 10 minutes or a full nap time. The opportunity to be in your presence and be lavished with love and attention will bring the older sibling back to a place of feeling firmly attached.

Remember that this type of transition is a gradual process. In truth, each time your new baby reaches a new milestone, whether it be starting to crawl, grabbing attention with his or her first words or managing to reach the toy shelf, it is another new transition for your older child. "Send it back to the hospital" is often heard in some form or another from a sibling. I encourage you to embrace the fact that sharing his or her most treasured provider and protector (you, the parents) can bring up many feelings of fear and jealousy. The best we can do is provide a safe space for a child to express these very big feelings and move from anger to tears. By doing this you support your child in accepting the infutility of the fact that he or she must share you and that he or she is still completely loved, safe and provided for.

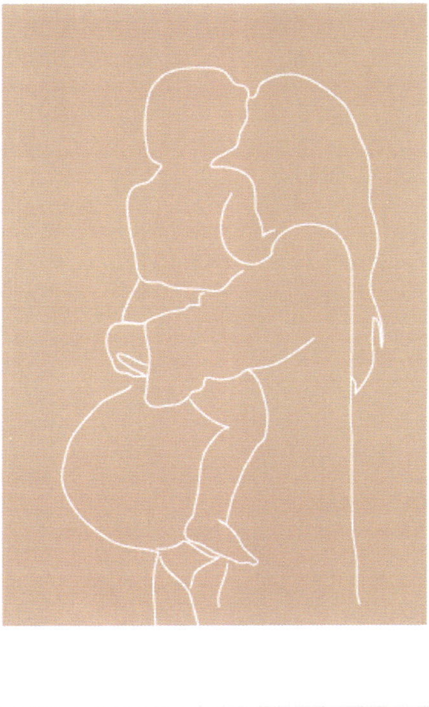

Bringing a newborn into a family with an older child can add a number of challenges to the family dynamic. These challenges vary according to the age of the child. Many of those disruptions can be softened by the timing of changes that need to be made, before the baby arrives.

TOP TIPS

- Try to move the older child out of a cot and into a bed a few months before the new baby arrives. This can help to prevent the older child from feeling physically replaced and may limit acting out through climbing out of bed or wanting to climb into your bed which they might not have been in the habit of doing.

- If you have decided to send your child to a nursery school or a childminder, introduce this change a few months before the new baby arrives. The older child will then be familiar with the routine of going to school and won't think that it is to free up mum to look after the newborn.

- Get your older child excited about the arrival of his/her new sibling. Talk about the new baby and let them feel the baby kick. Talk about why mummy might be tired or why mummy needs to rest a little more than usual. There is a wonderful book that can help you with this that is on the downloadable Shopping List. Buy a gift 'from the new baby' that you can give to your older child on the day that they meet them and talk about that gift before the baby arrives. You can even ask them what gift they might like.

- Once the baby arrives, try to include your older child in looking after their new sibling. Let them hold and touch the baby without shouting or cautioning them. Children have an innate awareness of when they might need to be gentle and babies are far more resilient than we think. The bond that forms between your children will then replace feelings of resentment that your affections are in competition.

- When bottle breastfeeding your baby, your older child might act out or feel jealous. It can be helpful to have a basket of toys and activities that you bring out only when nursing so that the older child feels included.

"No matter how much the older child may have wished for a baby brother or sister, the reality of this shift in the parents' attention and affection is felt as a loss"

- Janet Lansbury

TAKING CARE OF A NEWBORN

by Caitlin

Suddenly you arrive home and realize that you are charged with keeping this small, dependant baby alive. They can't tell you what is wrong and crying is the only form of communication you have to interpret whether it is sleep, comfort, milk, winding or a nappy change that will provide calm. Sometimes you will offer all five, more than once, and still the crying continues. Don't be too hard on yourself and be sensitive to when it is your own frustration that your baby is crying to calm. It is okay to allow someone else to give your child what they need at that moment. It does not make you less of a mother.

"A baby is born with a need to be loved.
And never outgrows it."

- Frank A Clark

SLEEP

Your choice on where your baby sleeps is up to you. It is good to be aware of the amount of clutter that fills that space and to know that they, especially newbown babies, are less able to move their heads away from blankets or toys that may cover their nose and mouth. It is ideal to have them lying with their feet against the bottom of their cot or side sleeper, so that they can kick up against it to push their heads up from under a blanket. You may find that your baby prefers sleeping on their side or tummy, having fallen asleep propped up against you. It is okay to lie them down with a support that can replace the position you held, as long as you can hear and see that their airway is open. Many parents are scared out of co-sleeping because of the risk that you will roll over and squash your baby. Breastfeeding mums' bodies form a natural 'c-curve' next to the baby which makes for safe co-sleeping. If you choose this option, make sure that your bed is big enough for each of you to have your own space. This is where a side sleeper is ideal, allowing a defined space that is right next to you to feel and hear your baby's breathing. If your baby has had respiratory problems and spent time in the NICU or you are particularly anxious about not waking up at night, you can invest in a breathing mat or an apnoea mat that your baby sleeps on. It will register if your baby stops breathing and sound an alarm to wake you.

GUEST CONTRIBUTOR | KERRY SECKER

Going to sleep is separation from you, and your new baby needs preparation for this. It's never too early to start a little bedtime routine for your baby. Doing 3 or 4 things in the same order in the run up to their bedtime helps them to anticipate what's happening. They love things to feel familiar!

Here's my suggestions for starting a sleep routine:

- **BATH** | You don't have to bath your baby every day but it lets them know bedtime is approaching and aids melatonin production. At your baby's age they need all the help they can get!
- **MASSAGE** | This doesn't have to be anything fancy but some simple strokes can help your baby to settle especially if wind/colic is an issue.
- Nappy and pjs
- White noise on
- Sing a sleepy song
- **BIG KISS AND CUDDLE** | It feels amazing and it also releases oxytocin which can help sleep
- Feed

You've probably been told to put your baby down drowsy but awake. This is almost impossible for your new baby, who's either awake or milk drunk. It's ok to help your baby to sleep by cuddling, feeding, rocking and stroking. You're not making a rod for your own back, there isn't one!

Your baby is born with a startle reflex called the Moro reflex. The muscles in their limbs and neck contract with a sudden movement, jolt or noise. This can disturb them as they're settling to sleep and sleeping. Safe swaddling can help your baby drift off to sleep and stay asleep.

If you do decide to swaddle it's important to do it safely:

- Only swaddle with light materials
- Keep baby's room temperature between 16 and 19 degrees
- Always place your baby on their back to sleep
- Make sure you leave enough room for their legs to move up and out for healthy hip development
- Don't swaddle whilst co-sleeping
- Don't swaddle once they can roll

Use the QR Code to visit the link to The Beyond Sleep Training Project to read about how to safely bedshare with your baby.

thebeyondsleeptrainingproject.com/faqs/how-do-i-safely-bedshare

BABY RESUSCITATION

It can be life saving to know basic infant CPR. If you are ever faced with a child that is not breathing you can run through these basic steps:

Hazards - make sure there is nothing that could have endangered the baby, like live electricity
Hello - try to wake your baby by talking and rubbing their chest
Help - call for help and for your partner to call the ambulance

A. Airway
Check their mouth and nose and clear anything that may be blocking them including something they might have tried to swallow. Be careful not to push anything further into their mouth.

B. Breathing
With your fingers, gently lift the chin bone and ensure that the airway is open with the head and neck in line. Look, Listen and Feel for 10 seconds for breath sounds by placing your ear next to the mouth and nose looking at their chest. Listen and feel for the breath sounds against your ear.

Give 5 rescue breaths by placing your mouth over their nose and mouth and blowing over them for one second so that you can see the chest rises and then falls with each breath.

Once there are signs of life (movement, coughing or normal breathing), turn your child to the side (recovery position) and continue to monitor until help arrives.

C. Compressions
Using your two fingers, press down firmly on the middle of the chest to compress it by a third of its depth and release repeatedly at a rate of 100 to 120 compressions per minute. After 30 compressions give 2 effective rescue breaths as above. Continue until help arrives or they show signs of life.

Click on the following link or scan the QR code to watch a short video on how to give CPR to a baby.

https://youtu.be/avYRvVHAvfM

Scan this QR code to view an infographic on First Aid for Baby.

www.eshn.co.uk/wp-content/uploads/2016/01/Essential-Baby-First-aid-poster-combined.pdf

FEEDING

You will experience a lot of pressure to breastfeed your baby. It is cheaper, more sterile, and gives your baby antibodies and the right balance of nutrients. More important than that, when a baby latches their mouth onto a mum's areola and suckles, oxytocin is released. This hormone, also known as the love hormone, promotes contraction of the glands and ducts that let down milk and also cause contraction of the uterus to stop the bleeding and to promote it coming back to its original size.

What a lot of people don't talk about is how challenging breastfeeding can be and how much it may take out of you. Your body has gone through a major trauma and is slowly trying to repair and recover its hormone balance, while simultaneously trying to make the nourishing elixir your baby needs to grow. As in pregnancy, your body will preferentially use all the nutrients it needs to make this milk at the cost of its own attempts at recovery. This leaves many women feeling tired, anxious and confused as to why they struggle to meet the demands of their baby's weekly weigh-ins.

Your baby only needs a teaspoon of the thick, syrupy colostrum that your breasts make in your baby's first day of life. While their stomachs grow, your breasts will meet their increasing demands when the milk 'comes in' on day three to five. This can feel strange; your nipples can sting with the let down and your breasts may become tense and full overnight. You might have so much milk that your nipples become like tiny smarties that your baby struggles to draw deep enough against their palate, to massage their tongue against the areola to push out the milk. Tongue tie, inverted nipples or poor latch can cause sore, even bleeding, nipples. Mums who have a traumatic birth or a caesarian may have a delay in their milk coming in. Breastfeeding takes practise. Establishing breastfeeding takes endurance, but it does get easier.

Fed is best. The ultimate goal is to ensure that your baby is fed. There is no harm in giving your child formula if your recovery or anxiety is making breastfeeding difficult. Engorged breasts can be drained through massage, warm water or cabbage leaves to soften and allow your baby to grasp hold of the nipple and latch. Nipple shields add a layer that can protect sore, cracked skin and aid latching, in the case of shallow or inverted nipples. Using baby safe nipple cream before and after every feed can help soothe a painful latch. Tongue tie can be released or snipped to allow free movement of the tongue to 'milk' the breast. Through all of this, it is okay to rather give formula instead or to mix feed. If this makes you less anxious and more able to engage and enjoy the time with your child then that is best. You cannot go back and have that time again.

Formula feeding allows you to share the demand of feeding with your partner. It is also necessary for mums with food intolerances and allergies. Some breastfed babies experience colic, diarrhoea or skin rashes in response to what their mother eats. Formula feeding comes with its own difficulties. You may need to try a number of different bottles and different types of formula before you find what your baby 'likes' best. It is also more likely to cause trapped winds and constipation. Do not underestimate the benefit of gripe water and other additives that can help relieve this. You are your baby's mother and, together with your partner, you can choose what you feel is best to care for your child and grow them into who they will become.

BIRTH AFFIRMATIONS

by Caryn

You can decide on a couple of mantras or affirmations as a tool to empower you to tackle unhelpful attitudes and beliefs that pertain to birth and motherhood. This journaling section will provide you the opportunity to take stock of where you are at, after completing the third trimester section, and to design your own mantras based on what reminders you are needing most.

Use this template to craft your own birth affirmations which you can cut and stick on your wall to help visualise a positive birth experience. You can reflect on these during pregnancy and labour.

Here are some examples of birth affirmations.

Trusting in my body's ability to birth

- I can do this; I am doing it
- Designed to do this

Pain management

- I release and relax
- I surrender
- I trust my body and my baby
- Purpose over pain

The potential of birth to bring transformation

- My body given in love
- I am present to the process

JOURNALING GUIDE TO MANTRAS

Write a short, punchy statement that you can use as a birth affirmation for the following topics.

A fear I have *(now write a mantra to release or reframe this fear)*

Knowledge I have to empower me

Trust in my body

Pain management

How I plan to handle each contraction

Tuning into my inner voice

In closing, take some time in a journal to jot down other insights you have gained after journeying through Part One of *Holding Mama*.

Mama, thank you for opening yourself up to this journey of being held and learning to hold yourself. You've got this. We would love to hear from you so please share your learnings and any transformative moments you experienced after journeying with Part One.

SHOPPING LIST DOWNLOADS

We have put together a few different shopping lists that for all of the different aspects of the journey of new motherhood. These are all downloadable so that you can access them while you're out and about. Take a look at the lists available to download and visit our website.

for baby

From furniture to toiletries, toys and all the other things, we have carefully considered the simple needs of having a baby.

for mom

As a mother it is so easy to forget to cater for your own needs. We want to make sure you have the tools to shop for yourself without missing a thing.

packing for hospital

We've kept this as neat and tidy as we can. Download this checklist for your hospital stay to feel calm and confident before baby comes.

You can also access these downloadable lists by visiting our website: **www.holdingmama.co.za**

"What if I break the baby?"
The other moms asked at an antenatal class.

I replied, "What if the baby breaks me?"

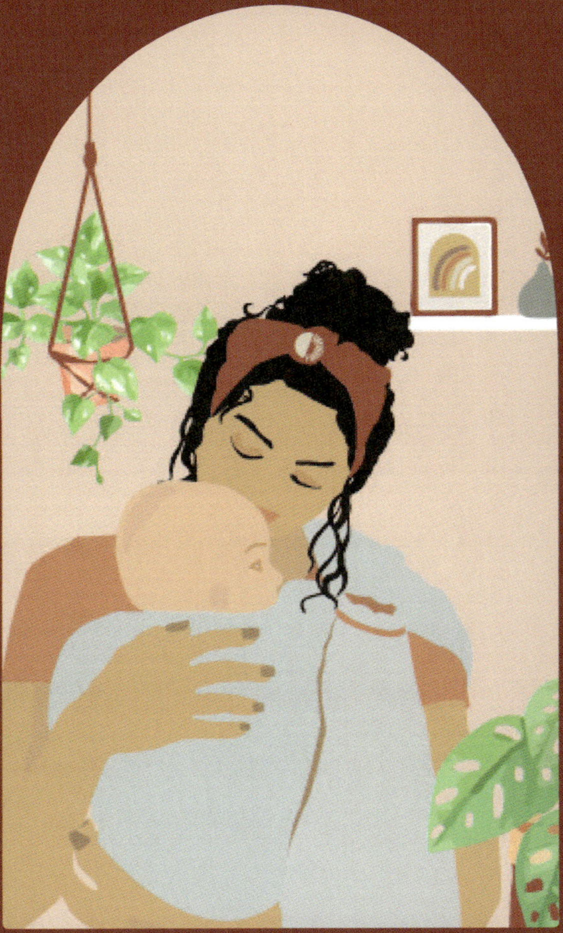

THE

Fourth Trimester

In grit and glory

My inmost being
where you were stretched
has formed my inmost being
as I form you
you form me
in a day
we conquered mountains
your head rests on your pillow
making roadmaps to
each other
and tomorrow
we do it again in grit
and glory

- by Caryn Edwards

INTRODUCTION

Congratulations on the birth of your baby. Take a moment to acknowledge the journey that has taken place. Months of physical and emotional preparation has gone into sustaining, nurturing and now bringing your baby into the world.

Many women experience the stark contrast between expectations versus reality - whether it's the birth you had imagined you would have, the nursery items you thought that you would need or the feelings of contentment that you thought you would have postpartum.

A friend of mine shared a very realistic picture of what it is like to be a mother when she described this memory from an antenatal class where a fellow pregnant woman asked: "What if I break the baby?" while my friend's reply was, "What if the baby breaks me?"

While we laughed at her witty response, there is something poignant about her insight - we do break when we give birth. We open up our world to both love and transformation that is expansive as well as having to rise to the challenges that, at times, feel like they have the ability to break us. Our world will never be the same again.

The truth about motherhood is that it reveals your innermost strength, slowly and surely like a muscle that was never used until now. You thought you were strong, but now you really know how much you can give, how much you can endure and how you can rise every single time.

Perhaps being a mother will be both the hardest and most beautiful invitation of your life. It's okay to experience conflicting emotions in all their forms - elation and despair, wanting to be close and connected; and wanting a break.

While you might be racked with questions, know that no mother, regardless of how 'qualified' she might be, has all the answers. If you experience doubt, guilt and anxiety in this journey - welcome to the club!

May this section remind you that you are not alone in what you are facing; and you will rise.

HOW TO USE PART TWO AND PART THREE

Part Two of Holding Mama will provide you with tools and information to hold yourself in the deep trenches of the Fourth Trimester and on the motherhood journey ahead.

This section of the book is designed to help you navigate a world of information by tuning into your inner voice in an effort to show you that in motherhood there is no 'one right way' - there are many. Your right way is what will serve you and your baby best in the delicate balance that goes into holding you as a Mama so that you can hold your baby.

Flip to the back and you will find Part Three which provides an opportunity for weekly journaling. There is one reflection for every week of the fourth trimester and questions for journaling. This is a valuable space to practise tools to help you in this time, as well as to document the early days of motherhood.

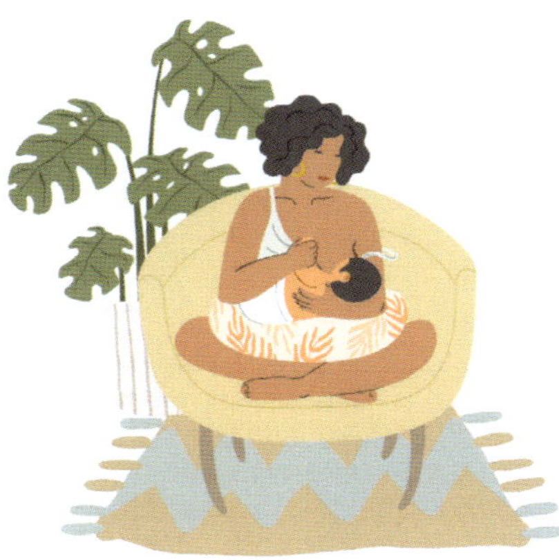

Motherhood is one way or another to break open

The way you give birth
does not determine
the connection
you will have with your child
or your success as a mother;

The way you give birth
is in one way or another
to break open
to a lifetime of opportunities for connection;
Birth:
the first of many breakings
Opening over and over again
to how much you can love

It is in being broken that
we are healed
Every mother bears the wound of opening to life

- Caryn Edwards

PROCESSING YOUR BIRTH STORY

by Caitlin

Many women come out of their birth experience feeling that it passed them by like a whirlwind. I can remember playing it back in my mind, desperately trying to retain every detail. What can be a beautifully empowering experience, can also be one filled with confusion and a sense of not living up to the magic you had hoped for.

Know that it is alright to feel joy, accomplishment, relief, regret or sadness. The range of emotions you are experiencing and the physical toll on your body both have a huge impact on your present reality. It can help to talk about it and to describe what happened to others or to write it down for yourself. Some find this less helpful and might take some time to feel ready to do this. It is alright to do things in your own time.

Mums are often criticized for wanting to share the 'gory details'. If you find yourself wanting to talk about it or ask questions then don't feel silenced, as it can provide reassurance that what happened was common or for good reason.

There are often a number of questions about why things were done the way they were. Some healthcare professionals offer 'Birth Reflection' consultations that allow mums to go through their medical record to discuss the different decisions that were made.

Use this opportunity to ask specific questions about why certain medications were used and what effects they may have had on you or your baby. Ask what prompted certain decisions to be made and to escalate care at a set point. It can be helpful to verbalise relief, regret or blame that you feel for choices that you made or the choices that were made for you.

There is no 'right' or 'best' birth. What is important is that your baby is born healthy with as few complications to your own wellbeing as possible. This takes into consideration your physical, emotional and spiritual wellbeing. Be gentle on yourself and allow yourself to navigate the magnificence of what you have achieved.

"Mothering can become a meditation; a deep mindfulness that is satisfying spiritually as well as physically and emotionally."

- Dr Sarah Buckley

REFLECT ON YOUR BIRTH EXPERIENCE

by Caryn

When you feel ready, you can engage with these questions for reflection as a way to process your birth story.

Write down your birth story. Feel free to write as much as you would like, to encapsulate the experience and document details you wish to remember.

It is okay to experience a wide range of emotions pertaining to your birth story. As a way to acknowledge them, you can use these key emotions as a guide to debrief any part of your birth experience that elicits these emotions. Jot down which parts of your story speak to these emotions.

- Joy
- Wonder
- Acceptance
- Peace
- Relief
- Hope
- Healing
- Hurt
- Anxiety
- Resentment
- Disappointment
- Guilt
- Confusion
- Failure
- Other

Is there a part of your birth story that requires healing? What will serve you best in finding acceptance in this area? For example, what support can you ask for? If it is helpful to journal about this area, use this space to acknowledge what is going on for you.

Mama, healing is not linear. Know that the memories of your birth can be triggering. Acknowledge the triggers as they come up and give yourself lots of grace.

MOODS & EMOTIONS IN THE FOURTH TRIMESTER

by Caryn

"Serious transformation begins with two commitments: the courage to try new things and act in new ways, the honesty needed to no longer hide from and lie to ourselves."

- Yung Pueblo

MOODS FROM A LIFE-COACHING LENS:
Self-Coaching and calming anxiety with curiosity and discernment

Know that every mother faces a myriad of emotions and it is normal to experience a level of anxiety and other moods. However, if your symptoms are more severe and you identify with the moods outlined by Caitlin in the next chapter, it is important to seek medical advice. Likewise, if you have even the mildest concern and simply want to ask questions to set your mind at ease, or if you don't feel like your usual self, speak to your healthcare provider.

SELF-COACHING

Regardless of what emotional experience you are having and what support you need, you might find it helpful to practise self-coaching.

In the practice of Ontological Life Coaching, we explore what dominant mood underpins the issue at hand. A mood and an emotion are differentiated by the fact that a mood is a sustained emotional experience, while an emotion might be fleeting. Of course, the way I refer to moods is different to what Cait refers to, in the medical world. It is important not to judge these moods as 'negative' or 'wrong', but to view them as helpful signposts of what is going on within you internally. So, take a deep breath and take heart! You do not have to suppress or ignore what is going on. When you take the pressure off feeling a certain way or trying to fix it, you will become more curious rather than judgemental.

In life coaching sessions with my clients, we explore how language, mood and the body generates one's reality and therefore if one wishes for a better quality existence, one needs to make shifts in all three areas. However, other shifts are possible too by simply acknowledging and validating the experience you are having, and by offering tools to help you cope. If this appeals to you, you can engage in the self-coaching exercise on the following page.

Identify a current challenge you would like to experience a shift through self-coaching.

1. What mood are you experiencing?

Examples:

Resentment	Frustration, lack of acceptance, feeling wronged or burdened
Resignation	Feeling demotivated, disconnected, unable to see how you or others can contribute positively to the situation
Anxiety	Feeling fearful, out of control, confused in the face of uncertainty, doubtful

2. What stories are you telling about this situation?

3. What language are you using in relation to yourself/others/the issue.
e.g. I'm not good enough, am I doing it right? Everything is dependent on me etc.

4. What language/story would serve you better? Reframe it by noticing what positive outcomes could emerge by telling a new story.

5. Imagine this new story. How does your body feel for making this shift in language?

6. What shift in mood is available to you now?

7. Carry this shift with you into your day and observe what happens.

Once you become aware of what mood you are experiencing, you will be able to notice the language (what stories you are telling about this experience) and how your body presents these stories and moods in your way of being and way of relating to the world.

Identifying how these moods play out in your situation helps you notice where this tension lives in your body and what stories are contributing to these moods.

The small shifts are the big shifts!

"A difficult emotion does not always indicate that something is wrong. In fact, it's often a signal that we're on the right track."

- Susan David

MAKING DECISIONS

by Caryn

THE TOOL OF CURIOSITY

There are many times in motherhood when I have wondered where my so-called 'mothering instincts' are. Why are some decisions so tough? How on earth do I find my voice in the myriad of opinions? How do I slow down to allow my voice to come to the surface instead of having a knee-jerk reaction?

These decisions range from how to get your baby to sleep, how to feed your baby, if and when you wish to return to work; and they can be downright overwhelming.

When facing a decision or uncomfortable emotion, the tool of curiosity will allow a gateway of possibilities to emerge rather than the tunnel vision caused by unhelpful thoughts such as "I shouldn't be experiencing this" or "things should be different". Know that difficult emotions do not always indicate that something is 'wrong'. Discomfort is a part of life; and discernment is making peace with the nuances of emotion and experience.

Becoming curious is gently befriending the decision or uncomfortable emotion and allowing it to take up space.
Rather than approaching it anxiously as a problem to be solved, allow it to simply be there. Breathe. Speak kindly to it as a strange visitor simply arriving with a lesson that will slowly be unpackaged. Don't rush to unpack it. You don't need to understand the lesson at this stage. You can simply know that every emotion provides information and you can choose how to best respond to it - whether that is acknowledging it or asking yourself how best to respond.

Becoming curious soothes the fear of failure.
Becoming curious is knowing you are not stuck and that you have options. It is acknowledging that there are many paths to take. The truth is that there is no one right way in motherhood. Often we approach an issue like sleep or feeding as an enormous problem we need to somehow figure out. When you are acting in the best interests of you and your baby, there is, in fact, no such thing as failure.

Becoming curious helps you to playfully try new things, to see the myriad of options not as a deadend of overwhelm, but a gateway to many options that you can simply try! You will find that an issue that arises is not a puzzle to be solved, so treat it like a game to be enjoyed where there is trial and error.

THE TOOL OF DISCERNMENT

The second helpful tool used to navigate decisions and concerns is the tool of discernment.

You will find your way if you "live the questions". You do not have to rush! You do not have to act on every trigger! Discernment is becoming curious about yourself and the situation as you seek to 'learn yourself' and any particularly difficult decision. It requires gathering the 'data' over time, rather than rushing to a solution. You will start noticing a pattern and you will be less reactive by being able to slow down your response. You will also be able to see the wood for the trees in your interior world - start noticing what triggers you and how emotions such as anxiety, joy and relief come up for you. Without having to hop on that bandwagon, you can simply let it become data, forming a bigger picture.

How does it look for you when you are triggered in your role as Mama thus far?

____

____

Similarly, we can discern the solutions we find for an issue. For example, Kolbe has recently been through a difficult patch of sleep. I have embraced the fact that we co-sleep, contact nap and that he is my permanent little 'cling-on' as my husband affectionately calls him. But I realised how our sleep situation needed some shifts to suit the family's needs. Constant wake-ups haven't been serving me well (not that they serve anyone well!) as I need to have energy for my toddler in the daytime too. I felt my interior world of emotion get very murky. After really enjoying the carefree bliss of enjoying my baby and taking everything one step at a time, I suddenly felt triggered to make some 'big shifts' overnight. I read the data on both sides - for sleep training and against sleep training. I felt conflicted by what seemed like polarising opinions. I suddenly mourned the idea of not having my little cling-on nestled under my arm at night. I so badly wanted to do what is best for him and best for me and it felt like there was no middle ground. And oh, the guilt that accompanies the many decisions where one is trying to serve both baby and mother and the family. I am a second-time Mama and yet I am different this time round, my baby is different and there is no-one-size-fits-all; and often, there are no clear answers. In the end, I found my voice and my way and it was worth wading through the 'data' and playfully using trial-and-error. I consider his sleep a big success story for me as a Mama not just because we are all sleeping well, but because I started honing into my elusive mothering instincts that became clearer and clearer as I sat with the discomfort and allowed the uncomfortable emotions to take their course.

"And the point is, to live everything. Live the questions now. Perhaps you will then gradually, without noticing it, live along some distant day into the answer."

- Rainer Maria Rilke

This is where discernment is essential. It will help you guard your peace. It will help you find your voice above the noise and the many opinions. It will help you pick your battles and make slow shifts. It will help you take this motherhood journey day by day and free you up with finding calm again to reassess tomorrow.

Discernment will give you a roadmap to your emotions, allowing the emotions to be signposts rather than guides - because not all emotions are very reliable guides! It helps you view your emotional world as a constant wave of up-and-down and to make peace with this ebb and flow, day in and day out.

It will help you make a decision not when you are at the peak or in the depths, but when you allow things to settle a bit. This is how you discern and this is how you find your right way.

JOURNALING QUESTIONS

What tough emotional experience or issue requires your discernment right now?

Name some of the emotions you are experiencing.

Write down what 'answers' you are seeking or what you hope to be experiencing instead.

Now shift away from the answers, and ask what are your options - to be playfully tested in the spirit of curiosity and trial-and-error.

Notice how your mood and body feel by using this playful approach. Write this down.

What do you feel is the next best thing for you to do here?

In the spirit of discernment and curiosity, can you allow yourself to handle this issue one step at a time today, and to reassess tomorrow? Describe what new attitudes and emotions are available to you.

How might this attitude serve you in your journey right now?

Remember that time is always on your side. You are never as stuck as you think. The options out there are paths to freedom. Keep experimenting, keep playing. There is no textbook about motherhood, but your one true voice that boils to the surface in the quiet of learning.

UNDERSTANDING PHYSICAL CHANGES AND UNEXPECTED CHALLENGES IN HEALING

by Caitlin

As with any physical differences between women; the strength of period pains, the fluctuations in moods and the length of labour, we all respond differently in the months of recovery. I have heard it said many times that the vagina is the most forgiving organ, erupting in ecstasy when accepting sperm, moulding and distorting to allow the passage of a new life, and then returning to its former inconspicuous state.

Society places an unfair pressure on women to return to their pre-pregnant physical body as soon as possible after birth. We are told to get up and get on with it as there is a new baby to care for, when any other medical procedure warrants days of convalescence to recover. Although there is much information on how to breastfeed, how and when to bath your baby and how and where to put your baby down to sleep, there is very little preparation on the changes that can be expected for yourself. That flood of blood when you stand for the first time after delivery, the first time you try to poo - fearing your insides might come out with it - or how to bath or shower around your caesarian or perineum.

Recognise what is normal and when you are feeling something that is impacting your psychosocial wellbeing. You know yourself the best and will know how you respond to feeling tired or unwell. You know how you usually face pressured situations. There are many things that will physically change over the time that you give birth.

BLEEDING/DISCHARGE

In the weeks after your delivery, you will continue to bleed out the blood that remains in your womb after your baby and their placenta have been born. The name of this blood is lochia and the amount that you bleed or the length of bleeding will be different for everyone. Often, mums that have had a cesarian will bleed less than mums who deliver through their vagina as the doctors have better access to clear out the placenta and contents of the womb at surgery. While it is normal for the blood to smell like blood, if you notice that it smells differently, together with dull tummy pains and general body aches, headaches or a slight temperature, you may have an infection in your womb. Blood is the ideal breeding ground for bacteria and they easily set up camp following all the interference and hours of labour. Women who have broken their water long before they deliver are at a slightly higher risk of this. Try to get to your doctor or midwife as soon as possible so that you can be examined and get antibiotics to clear the infection.

SCAR/WOUND HEALING

Similarly, for women who have any form of scar - cesarean, episiotomy or tears, these will usually take some time to heal and may go through varying shades of pink, red, purple and white. If you notice itching, oozing that crusts over, throbbing or the skin around the area appearing red then plan a visit to your doctor. Our skin acts as a natural barrier against organisms so when it is interrupted and manipulated it is less able to fill this role. Antibiotics started early will quickly clear the infection and promote better healing of the wound. Scar tissue is naturally fibrous and inelastic. This is very different to the tissue that was there before the scar. To promote elasticity, it is a good idea to massage the scar tissue as soon as it is sealed completely. Don't try to do this too soon as you can interrupt the initial healing and the tissues coming together and closing. Once you are certain the wound is healed, roll the scar between your fingers using a massage oil. Pull it up and away from the tissue that it covers to gently separate any adhesions that may be forming. In circular motions, massage the scar tissue to loosen those inelastic fibres. Some people's bodies produce thicker, slightly darker scar tissue than others called keloid. There are some options that are available to aid repair and promote collagen and elasticity such as Carboxy therapy and Platelet Rich Plasma (PRP).

MOOD SYMPTOMS

The high levels of progesterone, that have been maintaining your pregnancy, drop suddenly once you deliver the placenta and this relative deficiency leaves you feeling low and anxious. Progesterone is the maternal hormone that has a soothing, calming and relaxing effect on the brain. Together with the fatigue from labouring and the hours of being awake at night, this imbalance can lead to day three baby blues and, in those with a history of depression or bipolar, can trigger postpartum mood disorders. It is okay to feel overwhelmed at times or to cry from frustration, but when it is happening daily or affecting your ability to function, you need to ask for help.

These fluctuations in mood are not something that you can be expected to manage on your own. Talk to your partner, your mum, an aunt, a friend that is a mother or anyone that you feel comfortable with. Tell them about any dark thoughts that you are having and trust that it may bring you the help and support that you need to get through this time. Some mothers feel an uncontrollable anxiety that something bad might happen to their baby and that they must do all that is possible to protect them from harm. There is no need to be brave and do it all on your own. It is not always easy for others to recognize that you are not well, as they may never have seen you in this situation before. Men especially do not realize what is considered normal when adapting to motherhood and what is despair.

DEPLETION | NUTRITIONAL OR HORMONAL BALANCE

There is much that can be done to relieve these symptoms by looking into the possible causes. Blood tests can be done to measure hormone balance and levels of the various nutrients that contribute to our vitality. Imbalances in these blood results may reveal the depletion that you feel but struggle to quantify or explain. A low dose of body identical progesterone can be given to balance the deficiency and ease the symptoms of the transition from pregnancy to postpartum. Nutritional imbalances, caused by the months of pregnancy and labour, can be corrected with supplements or infusions. Iron deficiency is a common contributor to postpartum depression, headaches, fatigue, restless legs and hair loss after pregnancy. Thyroid dysfunction can result in restless anxiety with sweats and weight loss or depressed fatigue with weight gain. Any changes that you notice to be out of character to the way you would usually respond, should be discussed with a medical professional to investigate the ways in which they can be resolved.

HAIR LOSS

One of the biggest physical concerns that mothers share, but are too embarrassed to talk about, is the marked increase in the loss of hair. Hair is often the first thing that people see when they greet us, as it acts as a window into our physical well being. Progesterone allows our hair to blossom in pregnancy, growing thick and lush. Conversely, in the months after labour, the relative deficiency in progesterone and the subsequent imbalance can cause the hair to thin and fall away through brushing, washing and general day to day wear. Iron deficiency will usually develop during the first pregnancy and if followed by a swift second or third pregnancy, the body does not have enough time to recover the losses suffered in the pregnancy, labour and feeding of a child before being thrown into the cycle again. This can be the cause for hair thinning in repeat pregnancies and for noticeable hair shedding in the months after labour. Get your bloods checked and get in contact with someone who can help restore your balance of nutrients and hormones.

You may not know that your tummy will take weeks to lose the swelling of the uterus that accommodates your child. This came as an unwanted shock to me, when I was asked when my baby was due while he slept soundly in the car at a tender age of five weeks old. I was devastated that I was still large enough to look pregnant so long after I had delivered. It is normal to feel the very physical signs of being postpartum. Your breasts swell up, leaking milk down your front while you stand in hospital grade panties holding the thickest liners to catch the lochia that bleeds from your emptying womb. Give yourself the time that you need to navigate these changes. Be gentle and try to wear the changes with pride, rather than trying to hide every sign that you have brought a new life into the world.

COMPASSION FOR YOUR POSTPARTUM BODY

by Caryn

Pregnancy and postpartum can exacerbate the triggers regarding self-image and identity that you might already have had pre-pregnancy.

Even if you have a healthy sense of self-image, all women will bump up against learning to accept the physical and emotional changes taking place in pregnancy and postpartum.

It can feel unsettling. Questions such as, "Will my body ever be the same again?" or "When will I feel like my usual self again?"

It can feel scary - as any stitches take time to heal or limit your movement, as you lose blood after birth, as your breasts swell up in preparation for a function they have never yet fulfilled.

It can feel overwhelming. "Will my body ever be my own again?"

Navigating these physical and emotional changes might bring up the most pertinent question, "Why did no one tell me?" Many of these phenomena might be considered taboo. On the other hand, there is only so much that can be said and prepared for - the rest has to be experienced.

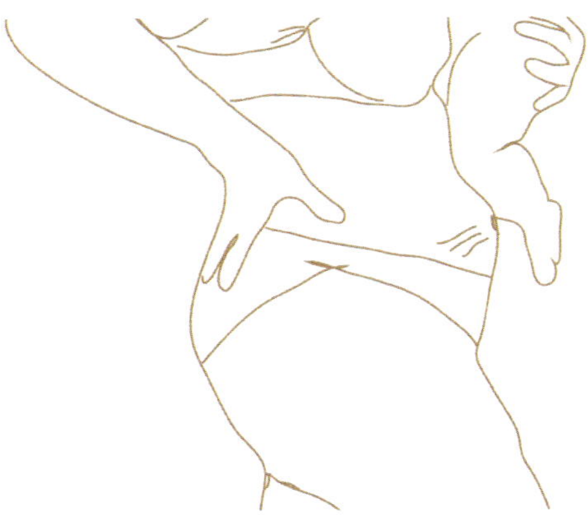

CARING FOR YOUR PELVIC FLOOR

by Jen Wareing

Where and what on earth is our pelvic floor? As a women's health physiotherapist, I believe it is the holy grail of our muscles. They're located in the base of our pelvis and have a few really important functions - they keep us from leaking body fluids, support our internal organs, support a growing baby and allow for pleasurable sex. Pregnant women are often told what a kegel is, but not necessarily how to do it properly - and that it is important to do pelvic floor exercises postpartum. We need to be able to contract fully and, probably more importantly, relax fully to allow for our pelvic floor muscles to work effectively with the help of a deep diaphragmatic breath. To do this: breathe in, open vagina and open anus as if to release gas, breathe out and close vagina and anus as if to hold any gas in.

As a physiotherapist with a special interest in pelvic and women's health, my aim is to provide a safe space for women to learn more about the changes their bodies are going through. In an ideal world, all women should see a women's health physio on a regular basis to check in with their bodies, become in tune with their pelvic floors and how they are functioning in the various stages of life. That's not always possible, so I believe it is imperative to have a postnatal 6 week check up with a women's health physio, as you do with your gynae.

This is not only to determine the state of your pelvic floor (regardless of whether you had a vaginal or cesarian section) but to manage and help symptoms such as prolapse, leaking gas, urine or poop, pain with sex, pelvic pain, to learn how to return to exercise safely, to learn how to manage a tummy muscle separation and so much more.

It has become incredibly taboo to speak about these topics and symptoms and, as women, we are so quick to brush them off and think that it is our new normal because we have had a baby, or because we are nearing menopause, or because we are ageing. It may be common to experience these symptoms, but it shouldn't become your new normal. There is help out there, you are not alone and you most definitely do not need to suffer in silence.

JOURNALING QUESTIONS

What aspect of the physical and emotional changes might you be having difficulty in accepting?

What stories are you telling about your physical healing/appearance?

What concerns might these stories be serving? In other words, what are your greatest cares and fears that they might be trying to protect?

Do these stories speak to any triggers you have?

Can you locate an area in your body where you are holding the tension of dealing with this pain point?

What standards might you be holding yourself to and are these standards accurate and helpful?

How might society and culture impact the standards you are holding?

How might having compassion for the pain point serve you?

What possibilities and invitations might this situation open up for you?

Let's refer to this trigger - be it emotional or physical - as your 'pain point'. The following questions for journaling will give you the space to check in with how you are coping with your changing body.

scan the code

for a guided meditation on pain points (also found on the next page) - by Caryn

Meditate

Carve out a quiet moment to slowly move through this meditation. Be prepared for the powerful impact it might have if you choose to engage with it wholeheartedly. Notice how you are feeling after working through these questions and acknowledging the pain point.

Breathe.

Place a hand on the area in your body where you have taken on the stress of this pain point.

Breathe.

Soften your body and mind to this pain by simply letting it be what it is. Now speak words and hold a posture of compassion. What would you like to say to soothe this area of tension? As you might comfort a friend, you are invited to treat yourself in the same manner.

Breathe.

Now mindfully acknowledge the invitation that this pain point poses for you in your reflections.

Breathe.

Notice any mind and body shifts that occur for envisioning this invitation.

If you feel comfortable, stand up and step into this invitation taking on the body of someone who shows and knows self-compassion. This is your tangible tool to live out the invitation and take on a new way of being.

In closing, write down any thoughts and observations after having completed this section.

EMOTIONS OF BEING A FOODSOURCE

by Caitlin

It is difficult to describe the emotions behind bearing the responsibility of nourishing your baby now that they have been born from your womb. When pregnant, we are mindful of what we eat and the various pressures we put on our body, in the form of stress, because we know that we want our child to grow in a calm, abundant environment. That mindset continues once they are born except that we suddenly remove our own wellbeing from the equation. Our baby will cry, strain or share physical signs of discomfort and we are tasked with interpreting that and providing the necessary comfort. What we cannot know is exactly which comfort they need.

This creates a constant uncertainty as to whether we are doing the right thing. Do I have enough milk? Have they emptied my breast? Should it still hurt so much? Could they have a problem like tongue-tie? Are they latching correctly? They have just pooed so does that mean they are hungry again? Should I let them fall asleep while feeding? Are they using me as a dummy? Is it okay to give formula to top them up? Which bottle should I use? Will this cause nipple confusion? Will this reduce my milk supply? Breastfeeding is making me so anxious that I would rather use formula - does that make me a bad mum?

A mum can run through a thousand questions a day, none of which have an answer that is right or wrong.

Bonding with your baby allows oxytocin to flow and that is what allows the milk to be 'let down'. But oxytocin is that shy hormone that requires a sense of safety and love to be made and is easily suppressed by overbearing stress. So many mums are desperately trying to fill a role they have had no training to learn. We expect to give perfection to our baby without creating a space to learn those skills of interpretation and comfort. I never expected that my son could suck a blister in my nipple the first time that he latched. I was shocked at how difficult it was to wind him and how imprecise it was to know whether or not he still had trapped wind. I was overwhelmed by how long I had to be awake each time I woke to feed him during the night.

There is no other combination of mother and child that is the same as you and your baby. You are a unit that is growing together and to sustain forward growth, you need to ensure that both partners are nourished. Food, sleep and support are the fundamentals of what you need to survive these days in the trenches. Your baby will grow to be able to talk and describe what they want and you will learn their subtle forms of communication but until then you need to allow a space for uncertainty. The greatest strength a mother can know is to trust her instincts.

CARYN'S STORY

Before giving birth to Sienna, I knew that breastfeeding might not be easy, but trusted we would find our way. After starting motherhood on the backfoot of a marathon labour and very little sleep, anxiety and exhaustion seemed to be contributing to a low supply of breastmilk. This, together with a painful latch, created a cycle of anxiety.

In that first week I was so physically uncomfortable that my husband would need to pass Sienna to me. I so desperately wanted to give her the milk she needed, but doubted that I was giving her enough and dreaded the pain of feeding so it felt like I was in fight or flight mode whenever she would wake from a nap, rather than feeling like my body could relax and I could bond with her.

What I didn't anticipate was how indispensable I felt. No one could feed her except me and what was troubling me was that she was not gaining weight. I wanted to persevere through the early difficulties of establishing breastfeeding, but at what expense? After five days, I woke up and acknowledged how desperate I was feeling and I called a mom friend and asked her if she had a stash of frozen breastmilk. Instead, she came to my house right after dropping off her three small children at school, brought me a tin of formula (to my disbelief) and her breast pump (and proceeded to wash my dishes right before she was heading off to work). I have never felt so relieved and supported. I had never anticipated offering formula and I was nervous to interfere with my supply, but I had arrived at the point of realising that my doubt and worry were probably not helping my supply and if I could just know that my baby was being fed, some of the anxiety would ease.

That weekend I set up an appointment with a lactation consultant. She assured me that my supply was good and she gave me instructions about how to increase my supply. I pumped, I used nipple shields, I took fenugreek supplements - I did it all! At the six week appointment with the pediatrician, I was told that my baby "looked like a lollipop" and that I needed to supplement with formula if she was going to gain the weight she needed. The doctor prescribed me a drug often given to help increase milk supply. I felt angry and conflicted. It's so easy to tell a woman to pop a pill. It felt like there were so many other underlying factors that contributed towards my anxiety and I was confused because I had been told that my supply was sufficient. The weight of making the 'right' decision and discerning whose voice to listen to made me question if I even had 'motherly instincts'. The simple act of feeding my baby seemed like a source of failure.

I took the Espiride, I offered a bit of formula each day, I continued to nurse on demand... I was told by some that I would harm my supply by adding formula, but I found my voice and found my way. It was the most tangible parenting lesson that there is no right way - simply my way.

Formula saved my breastfeeding journey. If oxytocin is the hormone responsible for helping my body relax and produce milk, formula was the buffer to my fear of depriving my baby, ironically allowing my body to increase supply. It allowed me to relax into feeding, it allowed me to know that my baby wouldn't go hungry and it took the pressure off me. It allowed me not to rely on formula anymore and to breastfeed for nine months which was a massive success for me - given that I questioned most weeks of the fourth trimester if I should continue breastfeeding.

I had come to embrace "fed is best" after feeling so triggered by the additional mental load of "breast is best".

Interestingly, my second baby has thrived on breastmilk from day one! It has been such an empowering journey, trusting my body and being surprised by how easy nursing has been this time.

There are many factors that go into the feeding journey and I feel that it is important to diagnose the underlying emotions and concerns and not just the physical difficulties.

Breastfeeding requires not only education, but emotional support too. It requires fostering a lifestyle of rest, relaxation and patience; and for a sleep-deprived new Mom, this can seem like an anomaly. If a mother wants to persevere through early difficulties, she must advocate for her rest and relaxation and be patient in the process. If a mother chooses to formula-feed for whatever reason, she must acknowledge any feelings of guilt or failure and reframe this into the success of feeding her baby. Fed truly is best.

JOURNALING QUESTIONS

What challenges might you be experiencing regarding being a food source (whether you are bottle or breastfeeding) for your baby?

Notice the emotions and where this tension lies in your body. Simply breathe and feel it.

What support might you need in facing these challenges?

If you find it relevant to your situation, you can come up with a mantra for feeding as a way of offering yourself compassion and reassurance. Write down a statement to which you can return in moments of doubt, anxiety or feeling triggered.
For example, "I take this feeding journey step by step" or "My baby is fed and thriving and that is what matters."

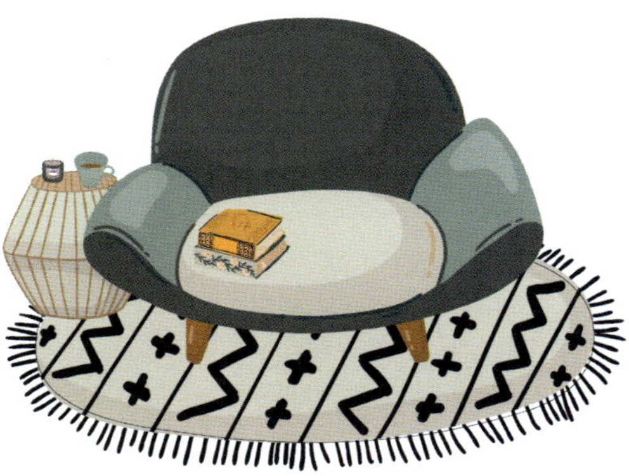

Motherhood is no-one-right-way

Honestly -
I still feel the tug
to do things the ‘right way’

To parent
To discipline
To put my baby to sleep
To feed my children
To do life
(The list goes on)
...The ‘right way’’

But what motherhood taught me
Is that there isn’t always one right way

I greeted the day in a hazy stupor..
But I showed up as a parent

I tried to be firm, I tried to be gentle
Perhaps I messed up..?
But I repaired

I rocked and swayed and walked and disturbed many-a-nap to get in the car..
But I put my baby to sleep

The pasta was picked out and the vegetables remained..
But I fed my children

That tug of rightness will pull...
The fear of bad habits chasing at your heels...
See it. Name it. Feel it.
Your breath loosens the tension

This is the tug of motherhood
Does it ever go away?
I think not

Can the voice of self-compassion soothe
The desire to do it right
I think so

You showed up
You repaired
They slept
They fed

Motherhood is days of no-one-right-way

- by Caryn Edwards

UNEXPECTED CHALLENGES IN BREASTFEEDING

by Caitlin

"Breastfeeding reminds us of the universal truth of abundance; the more we give out, the more we are filled up, and that divine nourishment - the source from which we all draw - is, like a mother's breast, ever full and ever flowing."

- Sarah Buckley

When attending antenatal classes we learn about the various facets of breastfeeding: how important it is to latch your baby correctly, the various feeding positions that you can try and the life giving contents of the milk that we make.

The reality, however, is filled with a number of questions that you had never thought of asking. How do I know that my baby has had enough? How do I know if the pain that I feel is normal or a poor latch? What can be done to assist in my experience of breastfeeding?

Breast milk is made under the influence of a number of hormones in the body but the contraction of the muscles in the glands and the little tubes that let down the milk is controlled by oxytocin. Mothers that have had a more difficult labour or a cesarian section may notice a slight delay in their milk 'coming-in' as their body recovers from the trauma of birth and the shy oxytocin slowly begins to flow. Similarly, babies that are born a little earlier than their full 40 weeks will be less confident in their suck reflex and may take longer to learn to latch and milk the dark areola skin around the nipple.

Our body somehow knows that there will be this delay and thus releases a thick, syrupy colostrum that is filled with a concentrated mix of nutrients. In the first day of life a baby needs only a teaspoon of colostrum to meet its needs. As their latch improves and demand increases, your breasts will naturally respond to produce enough milk to meet their increasing consumption. Skin-to-skin helps our bodies to tune in to each other and this together with a quiet, calm environment are ideal for a successful experience.

Our nipples are soft and sensitive and breastfeeding is quite physical. Most women experience a degree of discomfort in their nipples from the constant abrasion caused by latching and sucking. Invest in a good, baby friendly nipple cream that you can apply before, after and in between feeding. Nipple shields provide an extra layer of protection between the roughness of your baby's tongue and your nipples. Some women's health physiotherapists will offer laser treatment to 'toughen' the nipples.

Some mums choose to rather express milk and feed using a bottle. There are many breast pumps on the market and the choice depends on your budget and when you choose to express. Expressing takes time and requires patience. It takes you from a place where you do not know how much your baby consumes to being able to obviously measure just how much you produce.

I found that the pressure of trying to express enough milk reduced my milk supply to the point where I chose to formula feed while I was at work and breastfeed when I was at home. Be aware of nipple confusion and that your baby might choose to favour one method of feeding over another.

There are many differing opinions on dummies and whether they will interfere with successful breastfeeding. You will find that some babies use your nipple as a source of comfort in the same way that others will use a dummy or pacifier. Any source of comfort has the potential to form a dependence. The need for that comfort depends on your flexibility to be able to provide what is sought. For example, if you are required to travel long distances where you are unable to feed to soothe, then a dummy can substitute your comfort until you are able to replace it. It can be stressful to hear your baby crying and feel helpless. It is important to be aware that your baby may develop a preference for the pacifier so, before offering it, you need to think about your own feelings around that. Trust your instincts and know the reason for your decision and feel confident in that.

GEORGIE AVERY | *Breastfeeding Consultant*

For many mothers, the word 'natural' is deeply associated with breastfeeding; an intimate, almost instant connection between mother and child through the closeness of feeding. However, like most aspects of motherhood, the challenges of breastfeeding (and feeding your baby in general) are often overlooked or not carefully supported and many mothers find unexpected difficulties in breastfeeding leading them to question their own capabilities and the dreaded fear of failure.

Breastfeeding is a learned skill: both mother and child participate in a sort of dance: a back and forth of communication through touch, voice and the pleasure of warm sustenance (in the mother's milk), learning through one another. Breastfeeding, although Nature's natural way for mothers to feed and sustain their babies, can pose many challenges varying from physical difficulties either in the mother or the child, emotional or traumatic challenges of the mother, illness in either mother or child or a lack of support through education and help when difficulties arise.

The keys to successful (and even enjoyable) breastfeeding are patience, understanding (knowledge of breastfeeding) and support. A new mother should be assured of gentle guidance in the early days of breastfeeding by a supportive healthcare team. She should feel at ease to relay fears or even negative emotions associated with breastfeeding without fear of judgement or failure. The breastfeeding dyad is aptly named for the fact that it is made up of two parts: mother and baby; both reliant on one another and thus both of equal importance and need of care.

Breastfeeding offers a baby so much more than food: it is the most secure place after the womb where the baby is enveloped in the mother's smell, her warmth and touch, her voice and then of course, her sustaining milk.

Finally, breastfeeding is ideally not done in isolation; a mother must know she has support on hand for any questions or difficulties, perceived or real.

BONDING WITH BABY

by Caitlin

Through the change and all the physical recovery, you will need to find space to bond with your new baby. The signs are subtle and easily missed and many mums feel that they are giving all of themselves and receive nothing in return. Absorb every glance, every look of interest and every 'first'. Those moments when they fall asleep in your embrace or when they are soothed by the safety that you provide. The days that you learn something new about the type of person that they are and the nights that you dream of the person they will become.

Celebrate your successes: a bedtime routine or the grams of weight gained. Learn from your broken moments: hours of crying without an idea of the cause. Use them as a chance to remember this love that you have given. Try to be intentional with your time. Look at your baby while feeding and sing or gently stroke their hair. Talk to them while you bath them and cream them before bed. Read them a story at night just to snuggle.

We live in a time where we are used to instant gratification. Before we have children we are able to do what we want and arrange to have what we want when we want it. But babies break open this mindset and ask that we become a gift to others - even in giving up our last ounce of energy without the certainty that it will bring the calm we so desperately seek.

JOURNALING QUESTIONS

On a scale of 1-10, how satisfied are you feeling about bonding with your baby? Embrace whatever emotional experience you are having without judgement. It is important not to blame yourself if you are not feeling bonded with your baby. It is not uncommon for mothers to feel this way in the beginning. If you think that there might be trauma or baby blues blocking you from experiencing closeness with your baby, it is worth reaching out to someone to help you process this.

What shifts, that are within your control, could be made to foster closeness with your baby?

Notice the practices that might be hindering bonding (for example, ample time spent on your phone or getting frustrated if they are not sleeping). Again, without judgement, simply notice your experience.

Think of one or two things you can build into your daily rhythm to foster bonding. e.g. playtime before a nap or one feed without being on your phone or a walk with baby in the carrier.

THE EMOTIONS OF HAVING A RAINBOW BABY: A BABY BORN AFTER LOSS

by Caitlin

Some women arrive home with their newborn baby never thinking that they would ever reach that point. The road that has led them there has been bumpy and riddled with obstacles. When that moment finally becomes a reality it can be filled with anxiety. What other unexpected challenges will I face? You may feel regret that your other children have not reached this moment and feel pressure to match the demands that the future will bring.

It is not uncommon to find it difficult to bond with your baby. Much of the pregnancy is spent trying not to get too attached in case something happens and results in loss. It is a natural defence to guard your heart against a repeated hurt. When your baby is brought home, the unexpected reality is unfamiliar and in some ways not fully prepared for. This makes it challenging to suddenly form an attachment with your baby.

For some, the anxiety of pregnancy extends into motherhood. They are fearful that something unseen might be wrong with their baby and may wake regularly to check that their baby is breathing or that they wake up when they are stimulated. The pressure to care for their child is so much more of a reality because of what has happened before.

While mum and baby groups are a source of support they can also introduce pressure and a means of comparison. For those mums that are struggling, it is difficult to see other mums that seem to be sailing through those months in the trenches. It may also be triggering to see other mums with children that have the same age gap that they would have had if their children were alive.

Acknowledge what you are feeling and be honest about what you find challenging. Allow yourself not to respond in the same way that your family or friends expect you to. Ask for help through psychotherapy or life coaching to support you through the transition until you reach a more settled ground. Give yourself the time and space to strengthen yourself through nutrition, exercise and reflection.

A Series of 'I used to think'

I used to think

Before I was a mother
I used to think
New babies just ate and slept
Took all the books from the library
To put my feet up
Hold her close, just to hold her close

When I was a mother
I used to think
I might never enjoy it
No one told me
Holiday was a lockdown
Old life, old ideas,
New body
Nowhere to go

When my baby was a small baby
I used to think
Her naps on my chest
A rod for my back
Finally in a bed
Thought she would stay in her bed
Held her close, again

When I was a mother again
I used to think
I could never "enjoy it"
Like they told me
Prepared the room
To mourn
Old life, old ideas
Old body
Nowhere to go

I am a new mother, again
No one told me
I would be in wonder of
New life, new ideas
New body
Somewhere to go

He's on my chest -
Not in his bed
Safe through the night -
Not sleeps through the night
What if the rod
Makes Motherhood
A series of I Used To Think

- by Caryn Edwards

THE IMPORTANCE OF SLEEP

by Caitlin

One of the biggest hurdles in the motherhood journey is that of getting sleep. This relates to your baby getting sleep and also to you and your family getting sleep. Every person that I have ever asked has shared a different view and most mums biggest fear is causing 'bad' habits if they're supporting their babies to sleep or harming their baby emotionally through sleep training.

Just as each of us are different in the way we experience difficult situations, each of us are different in the way we feel comfortable teaching our children how to sleep. As our baby grows and learns new skills, their awareness of the world increases. They also move from a place of seeing themselves as the centre of the world to being aware that there are other people and things around them. Their own personality will also affect which methods they respond to best. Trust your instincts, Mama. If something doesn't feel like a good fit, then try something else. Don't get disheartened if something doesn't work or if something that was working before suddenly changes. Read up on other mums' experiences and try to find something that suits both your and your baby's personalities.

KERRY SECKER | *Sleep Consultant*

Your new baby is naturally nocturnal during their first three months. This is because in the womb, your movement during the day would soothe them to sleep. Then at night, when it was calm (and there's less chance of a predator around!) they would wake and nourish from the placenta. This usually settles all by itself once they've adjusted and sussed out night and day at around 8-12 weeks old.

Your baby doesn't produce melatonin (the sleep hormone) regularly, until around six months when their circadian rhythm is fully developed - only then do they start to produce melatonin on a set sleep schedule. This erratic melatonin production can also mean erratic sleep patterns. It can be tricky getting your baby, who's naturally nocturnal, into a nap routine. It's sometimes even more frustrating than taking their lead and going with the flow.

It's also natural that your baby:

- Wants to be near or on you constantly
- Needs constant movement to stay sleeping
- Struggles to sleep in a cot
- Wakes or cries the second you put them down

I promise that you aren't doing anything wrong, and your baby isn't broken. They've just spent nine months inside of you and life is a little different on the outside. I say nine months in, nine months out.

I always suggest following their lead with naps until 8-10 weeks when they've distinguished between night and day, making it a little easier to start a nap routine.
In the meantime, white noise and a sling can be a life and sleep saver.

Meeting your baby's needs at night can never be the wrong thing to do. Crying is always communication and your baby isn't capable of manipulation! Going to your baby if they need you at night doesn't spoil them or mean they'll wake up out of habit. It does the opposite; they trust that you will come, it gets their needs met and everyone gets back to sleep as soon as possible.

Some points of reassurance:

- It's always okay to go to your baby and meet their needs
- It's okay to make eye contact and reassure them
- Reassure them with a sleepy sentence such as "It's okay Bobby, Mummy Daddy is here. You're safe and it's sleepy time"
- Your baby is the manual and they know what they need.
- Change their nappy before a feed and/or only if it obviously needs changing. There's no great way of waking up your baby than whipping their nappy off!

More tips from Caryn

- When placing your baby down, put them down slowly and gently (bum first) and gently pat them until they're settled before walking away.
- To test if they're ready to transfer from sleeping in your arms to their cot, lift up one of their hands and if it flops down without resistance, it means they're fast asleep.
- Don't stress if your baby rejects their cot and ends up in your bed! Follow the safe sleep guidelines and know that this too shall pass.
- It's okay if all the naps happen in your arms. You can gently try to get them used to a nap in their cot for one of their naps. But if it's taking too long and you're feeling resentful, give yourself permission to shift back to whatever method of going to sleep is working for you and baby.
- Don't let the words or opinions of others make you feel judged that you're doing things wrong. Whatever gets you and your family the most sleep is the best strategy. Babies are adaptable and you're not creating 'bad habits'.
- If your mental health is suffering because of sleep deprivation and you wish to consult a sleep consultant, research their approach and trust your gut if their advice is jarring to your values and needs.
- Bath, bottle/breast and books as a nighttime ritual is possibly the best tactic as it signals to them when it is bedtime and they will rely on this tool to wind down as they get older.
- Don't worry about baby having naps and bedtime at an exact time. Rather, follow their wake windows and avoid overtiredness and over stimulation.
- Don't stress if your baby doesn't fit the norm of recommended total hours of sleep. If your baby is happy and thriving, it means they are getting the sleep they need. But if you are concerned, speak to your pediatrician or sleep consultant.
- Sleep training (and the methods you use) is a decision you make as a family. If something isn't working for you and baby anymore, you are making a good decision to shift things to meet both your needs.

NURTURING RELATIONSHIPS: CONFLICT & BOUNDARIES

by Caryn

Nurturing Relationships with a Partner

It is normal to have to 'find' each other again after the birth of your baby. Your life has turned upside down - your body, your sleep, your lifestyle together has shifted dramatically. Your partner might feel resentful about how much your focus has shifted to caring for the baby; and you might feel resentful about the many sacrifices you are making in contrast to your partner.

It is common for partners to turn 'inwards' and become isolated in their struggles when resentment arises or when feeling misunderstood and underappreciated. Conflict arises when a couple struggles to meet each other's needs.

Relational happiness is ironically found in giving. By focusing on serving the other, your needs will find a way of being met without you having to grasp. Success together is sharing joys and struggles rather than going through them alone. By validating the other person's needs, you are already heading out on the road to success.

Some key points to consider about communication and conflict:

- Both of you are having to adjust to your 'new normal'. Acknowledge each other's feelings as valid.
- Follow the guidelines of communication discussed in Part One. Notice any of the 'Four Horsemen' that tend to arise.
- Find ways to self-soothe when you feel triggered. Notice the physiological response and emotional flooding as defined by The Gottman Institute. Simply become conscious of this response. Communicate about each other's triggers in a calm manner and discuss what each of you needs to do to de-escalate conflict and to feel heard, accepted and supported.
- Requesting what you need is vital. Avoid assuming that your partner knows what you need. Avoid becoming resentful about unmet needs and rather work on being assertive and respectful when making requests.
- Be gentle on yourselves when you feel like you are triggering each other or 'failing' at communication. Commitment to improvement is a more realistic goal than perfection.
- Let's normalise relationships needing work like a garden needs watering. All couples argue. All couples have conflict.

- Commit to fighting fairly and learn how to support each other better. Know that small consistent changes are the powerful ones. Each time you step in the direction of respectful, honest conversation as a way to find common ground, so you rewire the neural pathways. The road 'less travelled' in the habitual ways you react, think and communicate will become the road you are able to take more intentionally each time you choose healthy ways to fight. It's never too late to choose this path regardless of how much you might feel you're failing!
- Start an upward cycle. When you're feeling unloved and about to go down a downward spiral, surprise your partner with an act of selflessness. Notice what happens.
- Write or speak affirmations to your partner to thank them for what you notice. Look for the good and remind yourself of their goodness if ever you face despair.

QUESTIONS FOR REFLECTION AS A COUPLE

What stands out to you most from the key points above? Why?

Of the 'Four Horsemen', which behaviour tends to dominate your communication in conflictual situations? (e.g. criticism, contempt, defensiveness, stonewalling)

What can you do to shift this behaviour?

Thank each other for three things (qualities and actions) you have noticed since becoming parents.

Tell each other one thing you love about the other.

Tell each other one need you have and one way the other can support you in this.

Ask for and accept forgiveness for what it is causing hurt and truly mean it and move on.

Revisit the 'Conflict and communication chapter' in Part 1 whenever you feel you need to get unstuck.

Tips to Finding Each Other Again

A practical tool for finding each other again is revisiting what makes each other feel loved. The Five Languages, written by Gary Chapman, summarises five key areas of giving and receiving love. Often we tend to give love in the way we are comfortable with and enjoy receiving, but it might not speak to our partner's needs.

Discover each other's love languages by taking this test.

Click on the following link or scan the QR Code to take the Five Love Languages Quiz.

www.5lovelanguages.com/quizzes/

- Commit to one action each day that speaks to your partner's love language. Write it down here and notice what shifts it brings.

- Choose a time each week to designate a date. You might like to have two dates - one for the purpose of planning the week ahead and sorting out admin so that these conversations can be contained and not leak into the time for fun and connection. Add this to your weekly rhythm.

As for a date to cultivate intimacy, ensure that there are boundaries around this time such as:
- Committing to this time and making sure it happens
- Not bringing up conflict
- Finding fun things to do such as using a 'date jar' suggested in Part One and taking turns planning it
- Asking someone you trust to look after your baby when you feel ready

Note that intimacy does not need to mean sex. It is okay if one or both of you are not ready to engage in sex yet as you are still finding your new normal of togetherness. Intimacy is any act of growing closer physically, emotionally and spiritually.

INVESTING IN YOUR MARRIAGE

by Bongi Hill

Two months into life with two kids, my husband and I realised that we were not in a good place. We honestly had no idea that we would have more love in our lives than ever, while at the same time feel a bit broken. We were both pathologically exhausted. We had not spent a full night in the same bed because at least one child had some need that needed to be attended to. It was complete chaos.

We have become aware that in this season of having two small kids and being chronically exhausted, we can easily go into survival mode and neglect our love that also needs to be nurtured. One night, my husband and I sat down and wrote down some marriage goals. We each wrote down three things which we want to do better and see more of in our marriage. Some of the things were deep such as 'communicate needs clearly' and 'acknowledge and show appreciation'. There were also simple and cute things like having regular make out sessions and holding hands more often. Romance is important, friends, but it does not need to meet Hollywood standards.

We now review these goals monthly to make sure we stay on track and update them as needed. I have no doubt that I couldn't have chosen a better person to do life with. He's the one I want to have by my side as we navigate our way through the parenting trenches. We're now five years into doing this and I can honestly say it was a game changer in our marriage. We're not in a marriage crisis at all but we want our relationship to flourish and be at its best. It's the heartbeat of our family. If you are feeling the knock of life with small kids in your marriage or partnership, I'd like to encourage you to be intentional about nurturing that relationship.

Boundaries by Caryn

What comes to mind when considering the term 'boundaries'?

It is a concept that can be reflected on in many areas of life such as having boundaries about:

- In whom you confide and share vulnerable details
- Switching off from work and heavy topics to engage in refilling activities, relationship building and self-care
- Choosing what media you consume and noticing when to shut out other voices and opinions
- Taking on others' emotional load and balancing it with your capacity to give
- Accepting or rejecting outside influences especially those within your support system whose actions and opinions might conflict with your personal values
- When to raise issues that will potentially cause conflict

QUESTIONS FOR REFLECTION AS A COUPLE

From the list before, which area stands out to you as needing firmer boundaries?

What might be the result of setting boundaries?

What resistance do you have to setting these boundaries? In other words, who and what have you been trying to protect by not setting boundaries?

Notice that by drawing boundaries, you are protecting your needs and values rather than someone else's. Often we don't create boundaries simply because we don't want to offend. Are you able to become curious about what you can do to draw boundaries, and therefore, enjoy a better quality outcome?

What next step do you feel you need to take?

Click on this link or use the QR code to watch a short video by ***Dr Becky at Good Inside*** on her top trick for holding boundaries.

www.instagram.com/tv/CN_NtWLHNpB/

LET'S GET BACK TO SEX

by Caitlin

Sex after having a baby is different from what it was before. You have been through something that is physical and emotional and some of the needs that are met through sex are being met by your relationship with your new baby. The love hormone, oxytocin, is released each time you cuddle your baby and think loving thoughts about him or her. This is a hormone that is released when we think any loving thoughts and when we share those intimate moments with our partners. Many women, subconsciously, have this need for oxytocin met through the day while bonding with their baby and no longer have that need when they spend time with their partner at night.

Physically it takes time to recover from the trauma of childbirth. While the vagina is the most forgiving organ, able to return to its original form after significant changes, it also bears the wounds of tears, cuts, stretch marks and weakened infrastructure. It naturally takes time for us to physically feel ready to welcome a thrusting falus into those recovering chambers. The first time can bring back the uncertainty of losing your virginity. 'Will it hurt?' 'Will I bleed after?' 'Will I be able to orgasm?' 'Will I cause any further damage or slow down healing?' These are all valid questions and depend on a lot of different factors. As with many of the changes of becoming a mother, give yourself time to feel the transition. Be open and honest with your partner about any fears you might have. Don't be afraid to use aids such as intimate oils to help with lubrication and to cushion the sensitive scars. If you are concerned about how your wounds are healing, don't hesitate to get them looked at by a professional.

Sex is a bonding act in a relationship that renders two halves stronger and more united in their efforts. When much of what we feel is what is left from what we give to our child during the day, sex can be an injection of inspiration and renewed vigor. Allow your partner to do what they can to show that they love you. Allow yourself to feel desired and relished. Reach that level of physical communication that transcends what we cannot find the words to describe.

It is common for partners to feel differently about engaging in sex postpartum. Stereotypically, the birthing partner might feel less eager to engage in sex due to physical healing and the emotional adjustment of caring for a newborn. However, this is not true for everyone. Embrace whatever you and your partner might be feeling and remember that intimacy is the end goal - not sex. Find ways to build intimacy through the ways you communicate, show affection, spend time together and make every effort to understand how this need could be met for both of you. If you focus on intimacy and growing closer together, the pressure and possible conflict of getting back to sex is likely to lessen if you both feel understood.

FACTORS THAT INHIBIT SEXUAL INTIMACY AFTER CHILDBIRTH

by Dr Mpume Zenda

It is important to emphasise that sexual intimacy is a spectrum rather than an event or one specific act. Sexual intimacy during pregnancy and post-delivery should never come to a halt. It certainly will change - research shows there's a positive impact relationally amongst couples who maintain intimacy and connectedness. The spectrum is largely defined by what you as a couple are comfortable with and are willing to explore despite the awkwardness this season may present. This can range from conversations both easy and difficult, laced with plenty of affection and kindness towards one another. Women who feel supported are more likely to respond positively to sexual cues. Do whatever it is that brings out 'your sexy'. The point is, sexual intimacy doesn't have to mean or end with penetrative intercourse, whilst not excluding it.

Clinicians will often recommend safe resumption to sexual intercourse after six weeks post-delivery regardless of mode of delivery and assuming no major complications. That said studies have shown that 89% of women resume sexual activity within six months of giving birth. Some studies indicate that at a span of >18 months after birth, women have markedly lower levels of sexual pleasure and emotional satisfaction.

Various changes and factors (be it physiological, psychological or socio-cultural) can influence a new mom's attitude towards intimacy, how long it takes to resume intercourse, and the quality thereof post-delivery. Here are some important factors to consider:

Mode of delivery. With a normal vaginal delivery, short term recovery is often quicker (with earlier discharge from a health facility) compared to a cesarean section. This can further be influenced by whether you sustained any vaginal tears - spontaneous or cut (episiotomy) - during delivery. Healing may take a few days to weeks depending on the severity. Tears or cuts would make it particularly painful to have penetrative sex. Take time to heal and remember that physical healing does not translate to being 'ready'.

Urinary (pee) and Flatus (fart) incontinence can be a source of great embarrassment, and the resounding stigma surrounding such issues makes it harder for women to talk about it and get help. The unfortunate ripple effect may cause anxiety to a point where women avoid intimacy all-together. If it's causing distress and interfers with your daily functioning, speak to your gynae/midwife about an assessment and a referral to a pelvic floor physiotherapist.

Bleeding is mainly experienced in the early stages post-delivery, but also watch out for the monthly period that will resume (sooner if you're not breastfeeding exclusively).

Pain will certainly send your desire, arousal and orgasm out of the window. Pain may be as a result of a c-section, vaginal tears or vaginal dryness which is very common as a result of the fall of the hormone estrogen. Communicate what works for you and what doesn't work for you or your partner. Discuss pain issues that are persistent and not healing as expected over time with your clinician.

Hormonal changes post-delivery or during the Fourth trimester can lead to a further decline in sexual function as a result of the sudden drastic fall of sex hormones which is very common. Very crucial to look out for are symptoms of 'baby blues' and postpartum depression during this phase as they may have grave effects if not diagnosed and treated accordingly.

Take note that **breastfeeding** may impact your libido due to the hormone prolactin that is increased with the suppression of the sex hormones. Cracked nipples and psychologically seeing one's breasts as sustenance for the baby rather than erotic sexual organs can be a turn off, but this is no reason to deprive your newborn of the much needed benefits of breastmilk.

Finances, as well as any other stressor, will cause more sexual inhibition, and whilst you can't avoid expenses that come with the birth of a child, financial planning can alleviate a load of that anxiety especially with the added pressure of the pandemic.

Psychosocial factors. Whilst it's a time of excitement as the family welcomes the new member, it can also be overwhelming with uncertainties, anxiety and possibly a fussy newborn. Drastic changes in a short interval can contribute to the couple putting their sexual needs in the backseat.

Focus on setting time aside for just yourself and your partner. Remember you will do well as parents when you are well as individuals.

Fear of falling pregnant. Concerns about potentially falling pregnant is another real factor that can thwart a couple's sexual life post-delivery. Speak to your doctor about a suitable and reliable form of contraception or fertility awareness method. Note that breastfeeding is not a reliable method of birth control.

Cultural customs in different parts of the world should be supportive and enabling for the new parents rather than oppressive. As a couple, communicate your feelings and needs to one another, read, laugh, cry, change diapers together, try to share the responsibilities. A healthy relationship encourages a healthy sex life. The support of a partner, family, and your doctor is imperative and buys you timeout for yourself.

The bouncing back myth. Please take any unnecessary pressure off yourself - being a mom is already a full time job. There is no perfect pre-pregnancy weight or body to bounce back to. Yes, pregnancy will leave you with stretch marks, a few extra kilograms, a sprinkle of cellulite and it's all okay! You have just given birth to another human being and that's a miracle that we should thank our bodies for. When we don't feel good about our bodies, we are less likely to show up in the bedroom in all our glory. Focus on eating better, get back into exercise, embrace holistic wellbeing and love the new mother in you. Confide in people you trust about your insecurities. Seek professional help from a psychologist, life coach, personal trainer or dietician. This is no sign of weakness, rather a form of self care. This is not the time to be a superhero.

Understanding the transition you've encountered adds great value and wisdom as you navigate your mental, physical and sexual wellness as a new mother. Your body is constantly speaking wisdom throughout this process - listen, be patient and work with it. With the guidance of your doctor or midwife, you will know when you're ready. Speak up and always advocate for sexual fulfilment in every phase of womanhood.

JOURNALING QUESTIONS

What are your current needs and expectations for sex?

Has your partner expressed their needs and expectations?

If this is an area of conflict, brainstorm what you might like to say in a conversation to help you both feel on the same page. Go back to the tools discussed in part one for engaging in healthy conflict. Choose the right moment to engage in conversation, use a soft start-up, focus on listening to understand and express your needs and expectations respectfully and assertively. You can journal your feelings here:

If you are finding this topic triggering and need to come back to it later, feel free to do so. Consider reaching out for support if you need to navigate this with an objective party.

Write down a declaration for this area of your life by stating what you know to be true about your expectations for sex such as "I express what I need" or "I am patient with this process" or "we might feel differently about this, but we can support each other in what we both need".

DEFYING SOCIAL MEDIA PRESSURES & EMBRACING MESSY MOM LIFE

by Caryn

I was on my way to fetch Sienna from school and I caught a glimpse of my reflection in the car window as I clipped Kolbe into his carseat. A big loop of unwashed hair was sticking out of my headband. I suddenly realised that in the chaos of the week, I hadn't showered for two days. My head was swimming with undone tasks and the pressure to be fully present to my kids while feeling like I really needed time for myself - or just a shower! Perhaps if I had scrolled social media at that moment, I would feel triggered by the curated Mom feeds of neat nurseries and artisanal apparel. I was not fitting that picture right now.

We intentionally designed this book to be an airy, uplifting, inspiring space to open to when your house is a mess, you're a mess and your soul, mind and body is in need of being held in it all. If this book is the only clean room you have in your house, the only short moment of sanctity just to hold you then we have accomplished what we set out to do.

We don't buy into the illusion of social media - the highlights reels that do not fully capture the mental load of being Mama.

Take some time to notice how you absorb social media and what aspects of it might or might not be serving you in your current headspace.

JOURNALING QUESTIONS

What social media content are you being exposed to?

How does it portray or fail to portray your reality?

What are you seeking when consuming media? Perhaps it is connection, peace or joy (explored in the refill section). Does it provide you with what you are seeking?

What are other avenues of meeting these needs?

What time/s of day do you generally access this content? How might checking your phone or googling for answers be serving or not serving you?

In light of this, what action or shift are you feeling most called to right now?

Examples of actions you could take:

- Regulating what time of day and how often you visit social media
- Filling your time with an alternate activity when you find yourself turning to social media to refill, numb or escape uncomfortable emotions
- Unfollowing accounts that trigger you

Knowing what your triggers are, so that you can critically consume social media, is important.

By all means, use it, but don't ever let the falsehood of social media steal the real, raw blessings of your reality.

Things Undone Can Wait

I caught myself telling you
sorry, I've been trying to be productive
while your eyes peep up from my chest
The milk is making you fat
A lady told me on the street

A poet said
"Motherhood is cutting off the fat"
The leanness of time
And the guilt of not texting friends

This won't last:
Your skin soft as butter
A mouth that wants to taste
Fingers that focus to unfurl

This can wait:
Almost everything
Except putting fish fingers in the oven for your sister

Maybe motherhood is designed
To be unproductive
The cries of things undone...
Because they can wait

- by Caryn Edwards

A NEW IDENTITY

In Part One, we acknowledged the challenge it might be to assume your new role and identity as 'Mama'. Now is an opportunity to reflect on how you are navigating this shift in the thick of the fourth trimester.

JOURNALING QUESTIONS

What aspects of this role and identity (and the responsibilities that come with it) are you finding most challenging?

Are there aspects of this new life in which you are finding some sense of appreciation and gratitude? Take some time to acknowledge this now. Savouring gratitude for at least thirty seconds a day is necessary in order to let it soak in.

Do you relate to the sense of mourning your 'old' life? What do you miss most?

What would your future self, who is enjoying some of these 'old' freedoms, tell your current self? Do these words offer some comfort and perspective?

Sometimes it is beneficial to simply sit with the discomfort without having to talk yourself out of it. If this is what you need, simply take whatever action it is to feel - whether that is venting, crying, journaling, being.

Being in the Fourth Trimester is like being in a cocoon of healing and meeting your and your baby's very basic needs. Don't expect too much of yourself as you learn your new role.

This chapter in your life will be stretching you in ways you couldn't have imagined... It might feel dark; but it will be a ray of light when you look back because there's nothing more beautiful than what comes out of transformation. You might be asking, "When does motherhood get easier?"

It is my joy to share with you that not only did I ask this question, but I did find that it got easier too. Perhaps 'easier' is relative. There will always be stretching and growing, but you as a mama will strengthen your resilience muscle.

What used to be difficult will become more familiar. As you rise from one challenge, you'll be strengthened for the next.

You will find contentment again, you will find your voice. You will make peace with the push and pull of conflicting needs and emotions.

You will find integration in your new life, your new self. When I reflect on my new self, all that stretching has been worth it and I would stretch over and over again for the ones I hold.

Let go of the guilt of finding things hard. It's not only okay, it is normal. We are in this together as we find our way. And we will rise - as we learn to hold ourselves, as we reach out to ask others to hold us.

Continually foster ways of being, practices and perspectives to hold you in each chapter of motherhood. Jot down some ideas here:

Being a strong mama is advocating
for your need to be held.

MAMA MANTRAS
by Caryn

Use these questions as a guide for coming up with your own mantras based on where you are at right now - mind, body and soul - and to bring closure to the insights you have gained after journeying through this book.

What are some of the key lessons you have learnt by journeying through Holding Mama?

How had you been feeling before starting this journey and how are you feeling now?

Sum up the transformation that has taken place after reflecting on the previous two questions.

Write a short, punchy statement that you can use as a mantra for the journey that lies ahead. Use this Mama Mantra to 'hold' you in all seasons of motherhood by declaring it over yourself whenever you need it most:

Rhythm and Rituals

WEEKLY PLANNER

- [ ] **REFILL**

Allocate a time for refilling your 'cup' daily or weekly.

- [ ] **REST**

Allocate a time to get some extra rest (if that's possible) by requesting help so you can sleep-in or share the night duty. Take note when you feel you're taking on too much and need to slow down and be gentle with yourself.

- [ ] **PEACE**

Allocate a time to ground yourself in meditation, prayer.

- [ ] **JOY**

Allocate a time for joy and fun daily or weekly.

- [ ] **CONNECTION**

Allocate a weekly date purely for the purpose of connecting one-on-one with your partner, baby and older children. Allocate a time for catch ups with friends and playdates.

- [ ] **ADMIN**

Allocate a time to plan for the week ahead and invite your partner to share plans with you. For example, slot in errands, meals, chores, social occasions and work commitments into a family calendar.

- [ ] **CLEANING**

Decide which days you clean and tidy.

- [ ] **COOKING**

Plan meals for the week ahead. Allocate time for dinner prep.

- [ ] **SHOPPING**

Allocate a time to shop.

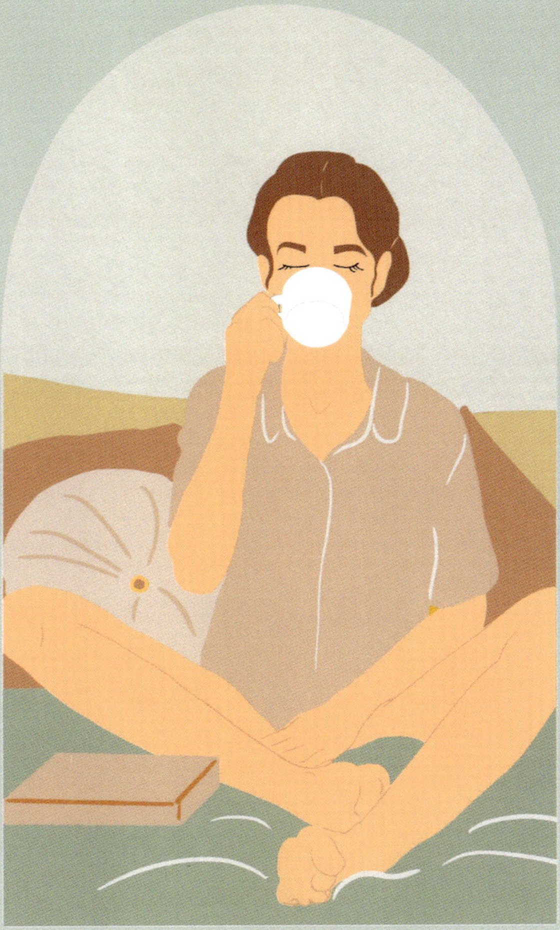

Weekly Reflections

A 12-WEEK JOURNAL

Enjoy the reflections. Let them speak to your unique experience; and if something is not resonating with you, give yourself permission to move on. I was once told by someone wise that some days just require a 'snack and a nap', and if that is you and you feel that the tools are just not 'working' today, listen to what your body, mind and soul needs. - Caryn

Acceptance

WEEK 1: **IT'S OKAY NOT TO BE OKAY**

As mothers we tend to put pressure on ourselves to feel good all the time about our children and about being a mother.

When I gave birth to my firstborn, Sienna, I remember describing the first week of postpartum in this way, "I'm not sure if this is heaven or hell". In one way, I was besotted with her, admiring the way her lips would move in her 'milk coma', the softness of her skin against me. In another respect, I dreaded the moment she would wake because I was experiencing such pain breastfeeding and wondering if she was getting enough milk. My body felt worn and foreign. Never had I been expected to fulfil the extraordinary task of sustaining a life while feeling totally broken in my own body.

That week I sobbed. I wondered if it would ever get better. What a contrast to the days leading up to labour - bright-eyed and hopeful about motherhood - to the shock of trying to hold my baby as well as myself.

When I went through the first week of postpartum with my second born, I could use that first experience as a reference point for how dramatically things do improve week by week, month by month. I was able to admit to myself that it's okay to not be okay!

If I could go back in time, I would tell this new mother that she can be honest about her feelings and that discomfort is not a sign of failure.

I would tell her to make room for all of it. Yes, it can feel like heaven and hell - and that is okay.

Can you take a moment to be honest about the tensions and difficulties you might be currently experiencing?

Breathe. Pay attention. Name what is going on.

Make room for all of it -
Emotions are not a measuring stick for your success as a mother.

Make room for all of it -
Conflicting emotions can co-exist.
You can grieve the old and find glory in the new.

Being honest is simply stating 'what is'.

Watch how things can shift simply by being honest.
Especially if you are not okay.
And from this space forward, take heart ***Mama, you will be okay.***

- CARYN

JOURNALING QUESTIONS

How have you been feeling this week with regards to mind, body and soul? *Simply naming the experience can lead to a shift as honesty and attentiveness to your inner world leads to growth.*

How does this week's reflection speak to you?

Based on your reflections above, identify one practical action you can take to move forward this week.

Turn to the next page to start planning for the week ahead.

Weekly Planner

Jot down plans for the week here, and insert your planning on the weekly calendar on the next page.

RHYTHM FOR THE WEEK

Plan in one thing that brings

- ☐ PEACE
- ☐ CONNECTION
- ☐ JOY
- ☐ REST
- ☐ REFILL

Are there any requests you need to make this possible?

TO DO LIST/APPOINTMENTS

	Date & Time	*To do/appointment*
☐		
☐		
☐		
☐		

MEAL PLANNING & SHOPPING LIST

The Week Ahead

MONDAY

TUESDAY

WEDNESDAY

THURSDAY

FRIDAY

SATURDAY

SUNDAY

Vulnerability

WEEK 2: **YOU'RE NOT ALONE**

You see the highlights reel of postpartum and motherhood:
Mothers seemingly put together at coffee shops,
babies fast asleep.

What you didn't see:
Bleary-eyed, waking up at midnight
Am I doing it right?
No matter the birth - we all bleed, we all need
To know we are not alone
The emotions of postpartum - the tears and the fears
To know we are not alone

Motherhood is a collective experience
Across ages
Across spaces
A body that is broken
And given up for a baby

That mother you see, 'put together' from the outside
But questioning, learning, broken - at times - from the inside
Is also you
Held across ages and spaces
To heal is the courage
To speak and to hear -
Know you are not alone

- CARYN

JOURNALING QUESTIONS

How have you been feeling this week with regards to mind, body and soul? *Simply naming the experience can lead to a shift as honesty and attentiveness to your inner world leads to growth.*

How does this week's reflection speak to you?

What shifts have you noticed since last week's reflection and journaling?

To be vulnerable with someone can help you know that you are not alone. To share is to find healing. There is a Spanish proverb that says - A burden shared is halved. A joy shared is doubled. Can you identify just one person with whom you can share how you are feeling? If this is what you need, have the courage to reach out to them this week.

Based on your reflections above, identify one practical action you can take to move forward this week.

Turn to the next page to start planning for the week ahead.

Weekly Planner

Jot down plans for the week here, and insert your planning on the weekly calendar on the next page.

RHYTHM FOR THE WEEK

Plan in one thing that brings

- [ ] PEACE
- [ ] CONNECTION
- [ ] JOY
- [ ] REST
- [ ] REFILL

Are there any requests you need to make this possible?

TO DO LIST/APPOINTMENTS

	Date & Time	*To do/appointment*
[ ]		
[ ]		
[ ]		
[ ]		

MEAL PLANNING & SHOPPING LIST

The Week Ahead

MONDAY

TUESDAY

WEDNESDAY

THURSDAY

FRIDAY

SATURDAY

SUNDAY

Patience

WEEK 3: **GIVE YOURSELF GRACE. EACH SEASON WILL PASS**

It's okay if things take time and things don't come easily. Take heart that every hard season is just a season. And it can feel infinite! Whether it's a season of sleepless nights, of rocking your child to sleep, of teething, of not having time for your partner or exercise or a hobby... Take heart that even if it feels like there is no end in sight, it is just a season. Retrospect will show you, but in the moment, you have nothing to go on. It is all new. It's okay to be fumbling around in the dark, waiting for the light.

Patience is a muscle, too. As you see one season end, you have the touchstone of that lesson to pass through the next one. While your emotions might be dictating to you - "It's too hard! "This will never pass!" - patience is the gentle, steady voice that says, "Just you wait... This too shall pass and you will be richer for it." Use every season as a touchstone for "This too shall pass".

The lessons I learnt in postpartum with each of my children are entirely different. With my second child, I now had the experience of enduring seasons to know that they don't last. What was a new challenge for me this time around, was watching my firstborn adapt to having a sibling. It pained me to see her 'mourning' the old, of not being able to make sense of this big shift and of having to share the arms that hold her. While I was able to hold the season of sleepless nights lightly because this challenge was already familiar to me, navigating her emotions was entirely unique. But patience, the muscle that is steadily built over time, reminded me that as much as I wished for her to see the joy of having a forever-playmate, I had to journey at her level, at her pace and by giving her grace, I have watched Sienna find delight in her little brother.

Give yourself grace, Mama. Pass through this season - at your pace.

- CARYN

JOURNALING QUESTIONS

How have you been feeling this week with regards to mind, body and soul? *Simply naming the experience can lead to a shift as honesty and attentiveness to your inner world leads to growth.*

How does this week's reflection speak to you?

What shifts have you noticed since last week's reflection and journaling?

In which area of life and motherhood are you finding it difficult to be patient? How might a patient attitude serve this?

Can you identify just one person with whom you can share how you are feeling? If this is what you need, have the courage to reach out to them this week.

Based on your reflections above, identify one practical action you can take to move forward this week.

Turn to the next page to start planning for the week ahead.

Weekly Planner

Jot down plans for the week here, and insert your planning on the weekly calendar on the next page.

RHYTHM FOR THE WEEK

Plan in one thing that brings

- PEACE
- CONNECTION
- JOY
- REST
- REFILL

Are there any requests you need to make this possible?

TO DO LIST/APPOINTMENTS

	Date & Time	*To do/appointment*

MEAL PLANNING & SHOPPING LIST

The Week Ahead

MONDAY

TUESDAY

WEDNESDAY

THURSDAY

FRIDAY

SATURDAY

SUNDAY

Self-compassion

WEEK 4: A SOFTENING TOWARDS SELF RESULTS IN A SOFTENING TOWARDS OTHERS

It is often easier to show compassion to others than to oneself. I share this tool with clients.
It is particularly useful when we bump up against our perceived failings. Self-compassion helps to reframe these moments as 'learnings'.

Kristin Neff, the thought leader behind self-compassion, offers a pertinent example of it at work in parenting. She was on an aeroplane with her child who was unhappy and disturbing everyone's peace. She walked with him to the back of the plane and while holding him, she focused on embracing herself and acknowledged the discomfort she was feeling. By attending to her needs and interior world first, she was better able to show up as who she needed to be for her son in that moment.

This example has stayed with me throughout my motherhood journey. It helps me acknowledge any personal triggers at work when I am navigating a difficult situation with one of my children. It helps me lean into that, to see the wood for the trees and then attend to their needs rather than suppressing my own. It illustrates to me the importance of not being a martyr to my own feelings and needs, but that my child and I are both richer if I am aware of what is going on within.

This tool can serve new moms in any trial - big or small - and as your child grows and you encounter new challenges.

Self-compassion is not selfish. It acknowledges that each of us is only human.
Self-compassion is not weak - it is learning to soften to the hard things rather than letting them harden us. The more self-compassion is practised towards oneself, the greater the capacity for compassion for others.

A tool to hold onto:
Kristin Neff's three steps of self-compassion invite you to speak to and comfort yourself as you would to a friend:

Step 1: Name the experience and emotion
Step 2: Okay the emotion - allow yourself to feel
Step 3: Know you're not alone - everyone suffers

It is often helpful to acknowledge where in your body you are feeling the hurt or discomfort and to place your hand on that area to practise loving touch.

- CARYN

JOURNALING QUESTIONS

How have you been feeling this week with regards to mind, body and soul? *Simply naming the experience can lead to a shift as honesty and attentiveness to your inner world leads to growth.*

How does this week's reflection speak to you?

What shifts have you noticed since last week's reflection and journaling?

In which area of motherhood and life are you feeling in need of practising self-compassion?

Here is a place to start - name the experience, okay the emotion, assure yourself that everyone feels like this at some point and you are not alone. Work through these steps slowly as you speak to yourself as a kind friend would.

Can you identify just one person with whom you can share how you are feeling? If this is what you need, have the courage to reach out to them this week.

Based on your reflections above, identify one practical action you can take to move forward this week.

Turn to the next page to start planning for the week ahead.

Weekly Planner

Jot down plans for the week here, and insert your planning on the weekly calendar on the next page.

RHYTHM FOR THE WEEK

Plan in one thing that brings

- [ ] PEACE
- [ ] CONNECTION
- [ ] JOY
- [ ] REST
- [ ] REFILL

Are there any requests you need to make this possible?

TO DO LIST/APPOINTMENTS

	Date & Time	*To do/appointment*
☐		
☐		
☐		
☐		

MEAL PLANNING & SHOPPING LIST

The Week Ahead

MONDAY

TUESDAY

WEDNESDAY

THURSDAY

FRIDAY

SATURDAY

SUNDAY

Connection

WEEK 5: **TURNING TOWARDS**

One of the key tools to keeping our nervous systems regulated is fostering connection with self and others. The same is true for your child and partner! They need to feel connected to you.

There are so many parenting methods and theories out there which are overwhelming. As part of redefining the 'metrics of success' as a mother and wife, I try to simplify and go back to this keyword - connection. If I am providing connection with my children in whatever we face, no matter how complex the situation might be, I know I am doing a good enough job. I might not hold all the answers, but I can at least strive to do all things in love.

Let's go back to your wellbeing - you are wired for connection. Motherhood can, at times, feel lonely and it is important to ask yourself what connection you can build. While it might not be possible to maintain a strong connection with everyone, you can foster it with at least one person on any given day.

Perhaps it is helpful to think of connection as a simple 'turning towards' rather than turning away when things get tough. Sometimes it is tempting to build a wall when we feel alone. To turn towards is any small act of opening ourselves up towards connection again.

Here are some ideas to build into your day or week when seeking connection:

- Take a couple of minutes to reconnect with yourself whether that's a check-in, some deep breathing and mindfulness, prayer or meditation.

- Focus on building in just ten minutes of connection with your child. Make eye-contact, create a window of being present amidst the to-do list.

- Connect with your partner for ten minutes. Make time to chat, use your 'date jar', play a boardgame, go for a walk, focus on listening and being listened to.

- Connect with your community - online or offline. Send a voice note, meet for coffee, have a quality interaction with the person behind the counter.

There will be times when you feel more connected than at other times, and that's okay. Motherhood is about finding yourself and others again, and that takes time. The small shifts - successes and progress - are, in fact, the big shifts.

- CARYN

JOURNALING QUESTIONS

How have you been feeling this week with regards to mind, body and soul? *Simply naming the experience can lead to a shift as honesty and attentiveness to your inner world leads to growth.*

How does this week's reflection speak to you?

What shifts have you noticed since last week's reflection and journaling?

How is the need for connecting showing up for you right now in life, relationships and motherhood?

What action might you wish to take as an act of turning towards rather than turning away?

Contemplate 'turning towards' and how this invitation looks. Spend some time in silence imagining what this looks like within your being.

Can you identify just one person with whom you can share how you are feeling? If this is what you need, have the courage to reach out to them this week.

Based on your reflections above, identify one practical action you can take to move forward this week.

Turn to the next page to start planning for the week ahead.

Weekly Planner

Jot down plans for the week here, and insert your planning on the weekly calendar on the next page.

RHYTHM FOR THE WEEK

Plan in one thing that brings

- ☐ PEACE
- ☐ CONNECTION
- ☐ JOY
- ☐ REST
- ☐ REFILL

Are there any requests you need to make this possible?

TO DO LIST/APPOINTMENTS

	Date & Time	*To do/appointment*
☐		
☐		
☐		
☐		

MEAL PLANNING & SHOPPING LIST

The Week Ahead

MONDAY

TUESDAY

WEDNESDAY

THURSDAY

FRIDAY

SATURDAY

SUNDAY

Time

WEEK 6: **IT'S A PHASE**

It might feel as though it will never end:
A baby in your bed
A bottle in her mouth
Rocking him in your arms
Years away from a Saturday sleep-in

Each phase: a challenge and a joy
Might feel like you've figured it out
Until the next phase rolls around

Motherhood has a way of displacing control
Showing what few constants there are
Guiding you to be more flexible
Grounding you in appreciation for small comforts

Each phase has a way of presenting lessons to be learned
Though the challenge might seem complex, the response is as simple
As being present to it and feeling the edges of discomfort
As loving in the way you know how

Retrospect will always show you
That no phase is as long as it seemed in the present moment
And that each is a touchstone of resilience
Giving you solace that if you could endure it then, you can endure it now

It might feel as though it will never end:
A cry that breaks the silence of night
A sick baby who will only sleep on your chest
Years away from independence
But retrospect will show you that time was but a slither of holding them close

- CARYN

JOURNALING QUESTIONS

How have you been feeling this week with regards to mind, body and soul? *Simply naming the experience can lead to a shift as honesty and attentiveness to your inner world leads to growth.*

How does this week's reflection speak to you?

What shifts have you noticed since last week's reflection and journaling?

What is a difficulty you are currently experiencing that might one day be a slither of time? It is okay if you simply want to acknowledge how hard it might be for you right now. If you feel inspired to approach it from a different perspective, imagine looking back at this phase as "but a slither of time". What might 'future-you' wish to tell you in your present challenges?

Can you identify just one person with whom you can share how you are feeling? If this is what you need, have the courage to reach out to them this week.

Based on your reflections above, identify one practical action you can take to move forward this week.

Turn to the next page to start planning for the week ahead.

Weekly Planner

Jot down plans for the week here, and insert your planning on the weekly calendar on the next page.

RHYTHM FOR THE WEEK

Plan in one thing that brings

- [ ] PEACE
- [ ] CONNECTION
- [ ] JOY
- [ ] REST
- [ ] REFILL

Are there any requests you need to make this possible?

TO DO LIST/APPOINTMENTS

	Date & Time	*To do/appointment*
[ ]		
[ ]		
[ ]		
[ ]		

MEAL PLANNING & SHOPPING LIST

The Week Ahead

MONDAY

TUESDAY

WEDNESDAY

THURSDAY

FRIDAY

SATURDAY

SUNDAY

Perspective

WEEK 7: **I DO IT FOR YOU**

In the early days of motherhood, it can feel like going through the motions - one nappy change at a time. There is little given back to you. Your baby cannot yet smile or show appreciation for the hours you spend meeting needs and having to stumble out of bed at unearthly hours.

In the early weeks of postpartum I had a moment of pausing from the mundane routine of it all and I looked into Kolbe's eyes and suddenly realised the obvious truth - "I do it for you!" It is easy to feel reduced to a milk machine or a human rocking chair. But the realisation of who you are making these sacrifices for, can shift the perspective.

A baby is not a project or a chore. A baby is a full person with dignity and needs. A baby is intelligent yet dependent. A baby needs connection just like any of us adults. It is possible to meet a baby's needs, it is possible to harness a baby's intelligence, it is possible to connect with your baby - no matter how young.

It is certainly a labour of love that goes into sustaining your vulnerable baby's life and you are not a bad mom if these sacrifices don't come naturally. It takes time to learn your baby's needs, it takes time to build connection and it takes time to appreciate just how remarkable it is that every act of giving to your baby is sustaining connection through the slow independence he is gaining.

- CARYN

JOURNALING QUESTIONS

How have you been feeling this week with regards to mind, body and soul? *Simply naming the experience can lead to a shift as honesty and attentiveness to your inner world leads to growth.*

How does this week's reflection speak to you?

What shifts have you noticed since last week's reflection and journaling?

In which area of motherhood and life are you feeling in need of gaining perspective?

Commit to one action you can take this week to pause and build connection with your baby?

Can you identify just one person with whom you can share how you are feeling? If this is what you need, have the courage to reach out to them this week.

Based on your reflections above, identify one practical action you can take to move forward this week.

Turn to the next page to start planning for the week ahead.

Weekly Planner

Jot down plans for the week here, and insert your planning on the weekly calendar on the next page.

RHYTHM FOR THE WEEK

Plan in one thing that brings

- [ ] PEACE
- [ ] CONNECTION
- [ ] JOY
- [ ] REST
- [ ] REFILL

Are there any requests you need to make this possible?

TO DO LIST/APPOINTMENTS

Date & Time	To do/appointment

MEAL PLANNING & SHOPPING LIST

The Week Ahead

MONDAY

TUESDAY

WEDNESDAY

THURSDAY

FRIDAY

SATURDAY

SUNDAY

Joy

WEEK 8: FINDING JOY & INTEGRATION AFTER BABY

You have just been born into a new role; and with that role comes an entirely new rhythm of life. Your time is not your own anymore - you are having to plan around your baby's needs and this can feel stifling.

I remember how having a shower was a really big thing! I had no family support with my firstborn so I felt totally indispensable - to the point that I felt like I could never have a break without feeling needed. My mother-in-law came to visit for a weekend when Sienna was two weeks old and I said, as I was going to shower, that if Sienna needed anything, she could open the door and I would run out to attend to my baby - wet hair and all! The expression of total calm on my mom-in-law's face suddenly made me realise how unusually panicked I was about meeting Sienna's every need and not being able to give myself space to breathe. I cannot tell you how free I felt in that moment to know that my unsettled baby was okay in the arms of another.

As time went on, things got easier and I began to appreciate small new freedoms as Sienna grew. In some ways it felt like I was finding myself again and becoming mindful of the ordinary and the mundane.

I remember the strange enjoyment of going back to work. I could go to the bathroom alone and drink my coffee while it was still warm. I remember the freedom of going back to the gym once a week, being able to turn on my bedside light to read because Sienna had moved into her own room, taking her with me to coffee shops to meet friends and relishing in the novelty of her drinking a babychino from a porcelain cup! Slowly it felt like there was a bit more space between us for me to appreciate her without feeling like I was losing myself.

I couldn't believe it when a colleague shared with me how she absolutely loved getting up in the night to feed her boys. It was a sacred time for them - no one else was awake but Mama and baby. I felt a little incredulous and guilty at the same time for not enjoying giving up my sleep!

Second time around, this need for my own space and freedom has been less drastic. I delight in meeting Kolbe's needs, co-sleeping, working from home with him. He's slotted seamlessly into my life - or perhaps I have simply become used to making sacrifices and being flexible.

I am compassionate towards that first-time Mom who dealt with the complexity of wanting to nurture her baby and be depended on and wanting space.

Whether or not this adjustment has come easily for you, try to accept whatever emotions you have around finding integration in your new life and new role.

Your baby will never be so dependent as they are now; and if you struggle with this, it's normal. If you delight in the cuddles, the closeness, feeding your baby in the sacred quiet of night - it's also normal.

- CARYN

JOURNALING QUESTIONS

How have you been feeling this week with regards to mind, body and soul? *Simply naming the experience can lead to a shift as honesty and attentiveness to your inner world leads to growth.*

How does this week's reflection speak to you?

What shifts have you noticed since last week's reflection and journaling?

In which area of motherhood and life are you feeling in need of finding joy and integration again? Simply acknowledge the discomfort without feeling the rush to change the situation.

Can you identify just one person with whom you can share how you are feeling? If this is what you need, have the courage to reach out to them this week.

Based on your reflections above, identify one practical action you can take to move forward this week. Perhaps this is seeking out a refilling experience as a way to add more joy to the week ahead.

Turn to the next page to start planning for the week ahead.

Weekly Planner

Jot down plans for the week here, and insert your planning on the weekly calendar on the next page.

RHYTHM FOR THE WEEK

Plan in one thing that brings

- ☐ PEACE
- ☐ CONNECTION
- ☐ JOY
- ☐ REST
- ☐ REFILL

Are there any requests you need to make this possible?

TO DO LIST/APPOINTMENTS

	Date & Time	*To do/appointment*
☐		
☐		
☐		
☐		

MEAL PLANNING & SHOPPING LIST

The Week Ahead

MONDAY

TUESDAY

WEDNESDAY

THURSDAY

FRIDAY

SATURDAY

SUNDAY

Celebration

WEEK 9: **CELEBRATING SMALL WINS**

Much of early motherhood is making peace with the mundane; and perhaps finding awe and wonder in the ordinary.

To live in awe is to pause and celebrate the small things - the house is a bit cleaner than yesterday! I was able to buy the groceries with my baby! I had an uninterrupted chat with a friend!

It is finding gratitude in an ever-shifting landscape of your baby's needs and development. The big milestones such as 'sleeping through the night' might suddenly be interrupted by a bout of sickness or teething. Motherhood is having an ever-expanding tool box of tricks to try - that work some days and don't work the next.

I had to learn that there was no end goal for my own comfort. I had to acknowledge that, yes, I have needs and would love my baby to sleep through, but I am not in control of this timeline. It is not a reflection of my mothering nor is it a prison sentence to my own joy.

These are practical things I did to find awe, gratitude and joy in the fourth trimester, and still do:

- I don't count my hours of sleep or embellish on how bad a night it might have been. It doesn't serve me well to focus on my tiredness.
- I always start my day with coffee in a pretty mug. It's a small thing but it inspires me to get out of bed, knowing that it gives me energy and a quiet moment to just be with my kids before the day starts.
- I appreciate friendship in whatever form it takes. Sometimes it's too hectic to get out and meet someone, but a voice note is a simple way to stay connected.
- I focus on the most important things in a day and let go of perfection and a rambling to do list.
- I let go of my own expectations for my baby's milestones whether it be falling asleep independently or counting how many naps he gets. If he is happy and thriving, I count it as a win, knowing he will get there in his own time.

- CARYN

JOURNALING QUESTIONS

How have you been feeling this week with regards to mind, body and soul? *Simply naming the experience can lead to a shift as honesty and attentiveness to your inner world leads to growth.*

How does this week's reflection speak to you?

What shifts have you noticed since last week's reflection and journaling?

Knowing that mastery and perfection in raising your baby is impossible, what would you consider 'small wins' currently? Well done to you! Soak in this achievement and consider this as success!

Can you identify just one person with whom you can share how you are feeling? If this is what you need, have the courage to reach out to them this week.

Based on your reflections above, identify one practical action you can take to move forward this week. Perhaps this is seeking out a refilling experience as a way to add more joy to the week ahead.

Turn to the next page to start planning for the week ahead.

Weekly Planner

Jot down plans for the week here, and insert your planning on the weekly calendar on the next page.

RHYTHM FOR THE WEEK

Plan in one thing that brings

- [ ] PEACE
- [ ] CONNECTION
- [ ] JOY
- [ ] REST
- [ ] REFILL

Are there any requests you need to make this possible?

TO DO LIST/APPOINTMENTS

	Date & Time	*To do/appointment*
[ ]		
[ ]		
[ ]		
[ ]		

MEAL PLANNING & SHOPPING LIST

The Week Ahead

MONDAY

TUESDAY

WEDNESDAY

THURSDAY

FRIDAY

SATURDAY

SUNDAY

Comparison

WEEK 10: **THE THIEF OF JOY**

Comparison is bound to creep into your motherhood journey at some stage or another. The friend of comparison is jealousy and self-doubt - even if it's just a mild dose.

It could look different for each Mom: envy of her smooth birth experience, or her curated Instagram feed showcasing the perfect nursery and family moments, of her postpartum body, of how much more sleep she is getting...

I once heard it said that "comparison is the thief of joy". Doubt about your mothering abilities or your baby's development will certainly be the thief of joy.

Everyone struggles. No one has it all together.

When you find yourself comparing, know that whatever standard you're aiming for is an illusion. Ask what it is that you are really struggling with and isolate it from the comparison you are making. Practise self-compassion in this area by following the three steps mentioned in an earlier section. By acknowledging what is really going on rather than giving into the victimhood of comparison and instead of trying to just sweep past the feelings, you will arrive at more authentic joy; joy for what is present in your life.

Practise the three steps of compassion now: Name it, feel it, declare that you are not alone because everyone feels this at some point.

If you are struggling with comparison, what is it that you are comparing yourself to? By acknowledging this, it can lose its power over you.

- CARYN

JOURNALING QUESTIONS

How have you been feeling this week with regards to mind, body and soul? *Simply naming the experience can lead to a shift as honesty and attentiveness to your inner world leads to growth.*

How does this week's reflection speak to you?

What shifts have you noticed since last week's reflection and journaling?

In which area of motherhood and life are you perhaps bumping up against comparing yourself, your life or your baby to the experience of others?

What is one true statement you can make about your life that reminds you that you are blessed and that you are enough? Gently remind yourself that no one has an easier, better or more successful life and that we all have our struggles.

Can you identify just one person with whom you can share how you are feeling? If this is what you need, have the courage to reach out to them this week.

Based on your reflections above, identify one practical action you can take to move forward this week.

Turn to the next page to start planning for the week ahead.

Weekly Planner

Jot down plans for the week here, and insert your planning on the weekly calendar on the next page.

RHYTHM FOR THE WEEK

Plan in one thing that brings

- [ ] PEACE
- [ ] CONNECTION
- [ ] JOY
- [ ] REST
- [ ] REFILL

Are there any requests you need to make this possible?

TO DO LIST/APPOINTMENTS

	Date & Time	*To do/appointment*
☐		
☐		
☐		
☐		

MEAL PLANNING & SHOPPING LIST

The Week Ahead

MONDAY

TUESDAY

WEDNESDAY

THURSDAY

FRIDAY

SATURDAY

SUNDAY

Unique

WEEK 11: NO SUCH THING AS A GOOD BABY

"Is she a good baby?" Oh, this is the worst question. I remember coming to the conclusion early on in my motherhood journey that this is more of a reflection of the ignorance of the one asking the question than it is of the baby.

What does it mean for a baby to be good? A baby who sleeps through? A baby who willingly goes to strangers? A baby who doesn't cry?

All babies have needs and express these needs through crying. An unsettled baby, a cholicy baby, a baby who only sleeps short stretches is simply being a baby!

Magda Gerber's RIE (Resources for Infant Educarers) approach asserts that all babies are intelligent, are full human beings and deserve respect. This approach has shifted my perspective in raising my children. These intelligent little beings are not capable of being 'bad' or of manipulating us. They simply need our love and empathy for whatever discomfort is causing them to need our arms to hold them.

Rather than viewing a settled baby as a metric of your success as a mother, remind yourself that babies have needs independent from your actions. It takes time to learn these needs, what the different cries mean and what their preferences are. View it as a success if your baby likes to go to people. View it as a success if your baby only likes to go to you. Regard it a success if you are still figuring out your baby's needs because it means that you are attentive to learning them. This is a life-long pursuit of learning that goes far beyond the fourth trimester.

- CARYN

JOURNALING QUESTIONS

How have you been feeling this week with regards to mind, body and soul? *Simply naming the experience can lead to a shift as honesty and attentiveness to your inner world leads to growth.*

How does this week's reflection speak to you?

What shifts have you noticed since last week's reflection and journaling?

In which area of motherhood and life are you in need of changing the 'metric of success?

What standards have you been holding this situation up against?

Create your own standards of success. Write down a few statements beginning with "I am doing a great job because..." or "I am a good mother/partner because…" Here are some examples: "I am doing a great job because I am attentive to my baby's needs" and "I am doing a great job because I am learning as I go."

Mindfully celebrate all your successes by naming as many as possible and savouring them in your body, mind and soul as you contemplate them.

Can you identify just one person with whom you can share how you are feeling? If this is what you need, have the courage to reach out to them this week.

Based on your reflections above, identify one practical action you can take to move forward this week.

Turn to the next page to start planning for the week ahead.

Weekly Planner

Jot down plans for the week here, and insert your planning on the weekly calendar on the next page.

RHYTHM FOR THE WEEK

Plan in one thing that brings

- [ ] PEACE
- [ ] CONNECTION
- [ ] JOY
- [ ] REST
- [ ] REFILL

Are there any requests you need to make this possible?

TO DO LIST/APPOINTMENTS

	Date & Time	*To do/appointment*
[ ]		
[ ]		
[ ]		
[ ]		

MEAL PLANNING & SHOPPING LIST

The Week Ahead

MONDAY

TUESDAY

WEDNESDAY

THURSDAY

FRIDAY

SATURDAY

SUNDAY

Chosen

WEEK 12: **YOU WERE CHOSEN FOR YOUR BABY**

At my babyshower, friends wrote encouraging messages for me to take into birth and motherhood. One friend wrote, "remember that you were chosen for your baby." These words stuck with me and still live with me today as I navigate a new set of joys and challenges in raising a toddler.

I return to the consolation that I have what it takes to surmount the burdens and questions that fall into my experience of mothering my children in their uniqueness. I return to the truth that each of us mothers have our own style, gifts and ways of showing love rather than falling into the trap of comparison. I return to the sacred mystery that somehow this beautiful human was paired with me so that we can teach and enrich each other's lives; and that while it is not always going to be easy, loving each other gives our lives deeper meaning and fulfilment.

There might be times when you doubt your abilities and decisions in motherhood. There will be times when you question yourself. There will be time when you wonder what the right way forward will be for parenting your child. The weight of these questions can be burdensome and can cloud the joy of the here-and-now.

So when you find yourself there, remember you were chosen for your child.

Despite your imperfections, you are good enough. In spite of your fears, you can show up. Despite not having the answers, you will find your way forward by returning to what looks like love in that situation.

How might the reminder that you were chosen for your child encourage you in this season?

- CARYN

JOURNALING QUESTIONS

How have you been feeling this week with regards to mind, body and soul? *Simply naming the experience can lead to a shift as honesty and attentiveness to your inner world leads to growth.*

How does this week's reflection speak to you?

What shifts have you noticed since last week's reflection and journaling?

In which area of motherhood do you need the reminder that you were chosen for your baby?

Can you identify just one person with whom you can share how you are feeling? If this is what you need, have the courage to reach out to them this week.

Based on your reflections above, identify one practical action you can take to move forward this week.

Create a final affirmation for the journey of motherhood ahead. Let it hold you in every season, Mama.

Turn to the next page to start planning for the week ahead.

Weekly Planner

Jot down plans for the week here, and insert your planning on the weekly calendar on the next page.

RHYTHM FOR THE WEEK

Plan in one thing that brings

- ☐ PEACE
- ☐ CONNECTION
- ☐ JOY
- ☐ REST
- ☐ REFILL

Are there any requests you need to make this possible?

TO DO LIST/APPOINTMENTS

	Date & Time	*To do/appointment*
☐		
☐		
☐		
☐		

MEAL PLANNING & SHOPPING LIST

The Week Ahead

MONDAY

TUESDAY

WEDNESDAY

THURSDAY

FRIDAY

SATURDAY

SUNDAY

CONCLUSION & ACKNOWLEDGEMENTS

Perhaps it was the pause given to us by lockdown in 2020 that afforded us the space and creativity to dream up this book.

Once again, voice notes over the distance sowed seeds of *Holding Mama*. We had no idea what form it would take or what the outcome would be, but we felt inspired to just start. We have loved every minute of putting this together knowing that if its words can find a way of holding just one mum or if just one phrase will latch onto the mind, body and soul of a multitude of mums, we have done what we set out to do.

We would like to thank the following people who have enriched *Holding Mama*:

Kelly Lubbee, thank you for being so attentive to our ideas for the look and feel of *Holding Mama*. You exceeded our expectations with the most beautiful illustrations. We hoped it would encapsulate the light and bright inspiration of a nursery for Mum. We chose you as our designer for creating designs that allow the reader to breathe - and your role has been vital in giving all our dear mamas around the world a 'room' to breathe. You have also been more than just a designer, but a dream-catcher and when we turn the pages of our book, we believe even more deeply in our dreams for seeing them tangibly.

To the photographers who provided us with our beautiful 'About the Author' photos. Thank you - Rozane van Heerden (@pose-a-rosey-photography) for Caryn's image. Thank you - Jonathan Boshoff (aka 'Dad') for Caitlin's photo.

Danielle Tennant, my own (Caryn's) Marmar, thank you for your invaluable insights and editing of the nitty gritties which is a talent, as well as for mindfully reading our book as a whole. What a privilege it is to have you so close on this journey - to pick your brain and for your ever-willingness to support, cheer us on and provide feedback. You continue to hold me as a daughter in so many ways.

To the husbands! David and Steven, thank you for enduring yet another conversation about this project! You hold the other half of this parenting journey and we are so aware that there is a big gap in our society for supporting Dads. We see the mental load that comes with fatherhood too and we appreciate your many sacrifices that allow you to switch between your many roles. Thank you for being our biggest supporters and for empowering us with the time and energy to follow our passions in supporting other mothers.

To dearest Bridget, who has enriched this book with her own experiences of motherhood through the endless messages and pages that she gently edited while juggling her own life challenges. I'm so grateful that mums get to benefit from your heart and vulnerability.

To the contributors - Charlene, Mpume, Jen, Holly, Kerry, Georgie and Bongi, thank you for filling in the gaps to our own questions. Your willingness to share your expertise and knowledge is invaluable and this book is a far richer resource for your experience.

To the Moms we have met - the Mamas who walk into the Mews Practice and those who have had online coaching. Your stories and experiences have inspired this book and we see courage and success in each of you as you own and share your unique story of motherhood.

To our dear reader, may these pages affirm the beauty of who you are and the fact that you were chosen for your baby. May this book inspire you with awe for your own story in the making. Reflect on it often, cherish it, celebrate it - and perhaps write it down on these pages.

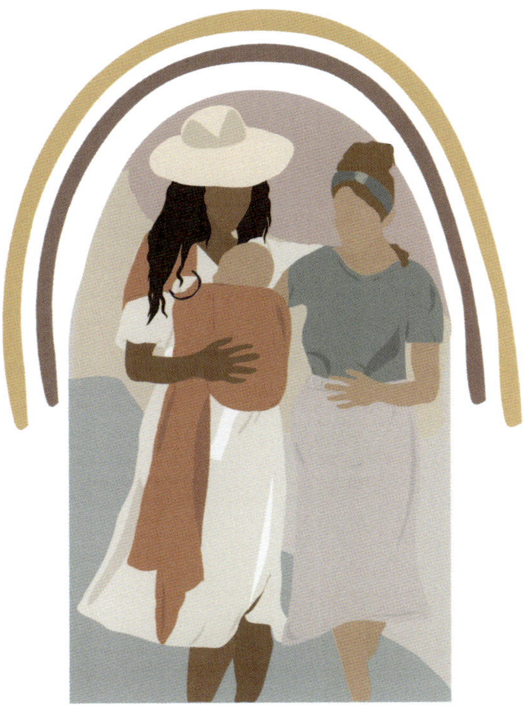

Printed in Great Britain
by Amazon

65716715R00104